ADVANCES IN

Vascular Surgery

VOLUME 8

ADVANCES IN

Vascular Surgery

VOLUMES 1 THROUGH 5 (OUT OF PRINT)

VOLUME 6

ADVANCES IN

Vascular Surgery

VOLUME 8

Editor-in-Chief
Anthony D. Whittemore, MD
Chief Medical Officer, Chief, Division of Vascular Surgery, Brigham and Women's Hospital; Professor of Surgery, Harvard Medical School, Boston, Massachusetts

Associate Editors
Dennis F. Bandyk, MD
Professor of Surgery; Director, Vascular Surgery Division, University of South Florida College of Medicine, Tampa

Jack L. Cronenwett, MD
Professor of Surgery, Dartmouth Medical School; Chief, Section of Vascular Surgery, Dartmouth–Hitchcock Medical Center, Lebanon, New Hampshire

Norman Hertzer, MD
Department of Vascular Surgery, Cleveland Clinic Foundation, Cleveland, Ohio

Rodney A. White, MD
Professor of Surgery, University of California at Los Angeles School of Medicine; Chief of Vascular Surgery, Associate Chairman, Department of Surgery, Harbor–University of California at Los Angeles Medical Center, Torrance

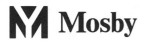 Mosby

Ⲙ Mosby

Publisher: Susan Patterson
Developmental Editor: Karen Moehlman
Manager, Periodical Editing: Kirk Swearingen
Production Editor: Amanda Maguire
Project Supervisor, Production: Joy Moore
Composition Specialist, Production: Karie House
Illustrations and Permissions Coordinator: Phyllis K. Thompson

Printed in the United States of America
Printing/binding by The Maple-Vail Book Manufacturing Group

Editorial Office:
Mosby, Inc.
11830 Westline Industrial Drive
St. Louis, MO 63146
Customer Service: periodical.service@mosby.com
                  www.mosby.com/periodicals

International Standard Serial Number: 1069-7292
International Standard Book Number: 0-8151-2732-4

Contributors

Ahmed M. Abou-Zamzam, Jr, MD
Fellow, Division of Vascular Surgery, Oregon Health Sciences University, Portland

Anthony J. Avino, MD
Fellow, Division of Vascular Surgery, University of South Florida College of Medicine, Tampa

Maseer A. Bade, MD
Research Fellow in Vascular Surgery, Montefiore Medical Center, New York, New York

Dennis F. Bandyk, MD
Professor of Surgery, Division of Vascular Surgery, University of South Florida College of Medicine, Tampa

B. Timothy Baxter, MD
Professor of Surgery, Department of Surgery, University of Nebraska Medical Center, Omaha

Joshua A. Beckman, MD
Instructor of Medicine, Harvard Medical School; Associate Attending, Vascular Medicine Section, Cardiovascular Division, Department of Medicine, Brigham and Women's Hospital, Boston, Massachusetts

Charles F. Bratton, MD
Chief Surgical Resident, Department of Surgery, Boston Medical Center, Boston University School of Medicine, Boston, Massachusetts

Edward B. Dietrich, MD
Medical Director, Arizona Heart Institute and Arizona Heart Hospital, Phoenix

Albert G. Hakaim, MD
Associate Professor of Surgery, Mayo Medical School, Director, Endovascular Surgery, St. Luke's Hospital, Jacksonville, Florida

Larry H. Hollier, MD
Julius H. Jacobson II, MD, Professor of Vascular Surgery, Mount Sinai School of Medicine, Chairman, Department of Surgery, Mount Sinai Medical Center, New York, New York

Brad L. Johnson, MD
Assistant Professor of Surgery, Division of Vascular Surgery, University of South Florida College of Medicine, Tampa

Blair A. Keagy, MD
Professor and Chief, Department of Surgery, Division of Vascular
Surgery, University of North Carolina at Chapel Hill School of Medicine

Jeffrey W. Kronson, MD, MSc
Fellow, Section of Vascular Surgery, Department of Cardiovascular
Thoracic Surgery, Rush-Presbyterian-St. Luke's Medical Center, Chicago,
Illinois

Glenn M. LaMuraglia, MD
Associate Professor of Surgery, Massachusetts General Hospital, Harvard
Medical School, Boston

Gregory J. Landry, MD
Assistant Professor of Surgery, Division of Vascular Surgery, Oregon
Health Sciences University, Portland

Kathleen M. Lewis
Research Fellow, Department of Surgery, University of Nebraska Medical
Center, Omaha

Michael L. Marin, MD
Henry Kaufmann Professor of Vascular Surgery, Professor of Surgery,
Mount Sinai School of Medicine; Director, Endovascular Surgical
Development Program, Mount Sinai Medical Center, New York, New York

William A. Marston, MD
Assistant Professor of Surgery, Department of Surgery, Division of Vascular
Surgery, University of North Carolina at Chapel Hill School of Medicine

Walter J. McCarthy, MD, MS epi
Associate Professor of Surgery, Rush Medical College; Chief, Section of
Vascular Surgery, Department of Cardiovascular Thoracic Surgery, Rush-
Presbyterian-St. Luke's Medical Center; Chief, Division of Vascular
Surgery, Cook County Hospital, Chicago, Illinois

Louis M. Messina, MD
Professor of Surgery, Chief, Division of Vascular Surgery, University of
California, San Francisco

Joseph L. Mills, Sr, MD
Professor of Surgery, University of Arizona; Chief, Section of Vascular
Surgery, University Medical Center, Tucson

Gregory L. Moneta, MD
Professor of Surgery, Division of Vascular Surgery, Oregon Health
Sciences University, Portland

Alexander D. Nicoloff, MD
Fellow, Division of Vascular Surgery, Oregon Health Sciences University,
Portland

Giuseppe R. Nigri, MD
Research Fellow in Vascular Surgery, Massachusetts General Hospital, Harvard Medical School, Boston

Takao Ohki, MD
Assistant Professor of Surgery, Albert Einstein College of Medicine; Chief, Endovascular Program, Montefiore Medical Center, New York, New York

W. Andrew Oldenburg, MD
Assistant Professor of Surgery, Mayo Medical School; Head, Section of Vascular Surgery, St. Luke's Hospital, Jacksonville, Florida

Kenneth Ouriel, MD
Chairman, Department of Vascular Surgery, The Cleveland Clinic Foundation, Cleveland, Ohio

Lewis V. Owens, MD
Vascular Surgery Fellow, Department of Surgery, Division of Vascular Surgery, University of North Carolina at Chapel Hill School of Medicine

Michael A. Peck, MD
Senior Resident in General Surgery, Department of Surgery, University of California, Irvine

John M. Porter, MD
Professor of Surgery, Head, Division of Vascular Surgery, Oregon Health Sciences University, Portland

Jason P. Rehm, MD
Resident, Department of Surgery, University of Nebraska Medical Center, Omaha

Linda Reilly, MD
Professor of Surgery, University of California, San Francisco

Lloyd M. Taylor, Jr, MD
Professor of Surgery, Division of Vascular Surgery, Oregon Health Sciences University, Portland

Frank J. Veith, MD
Professor of Surgery, Albert Einstein College of Medicine; Chief, Vascular Surgical Services, Montefiore Medical Center, New York, New York

Michael T. Watkins, MD
Associate Professor of Surgery, Departments of Surgery, Pathology, and Laboratory Medicine, Boston University School of Medicine; Co-chief of Surgical Services, VAMC Boston, Boston, Massachusetts

Samuel E. Wilson, MD
Professor and Chair, Department of Surgery, University of California, Irvine

Christopher L. Wixon, MD
Clinical Fellow, University of Arizona, University Medical Center, Tucson

Jay S. Yadav, MD
Associate Professor of Medicine, Ohio State University, Cleveland; Director, Carotid Interventions, The Cleveland Clinic Foundation, Cleveland, Ohio

Lu Zhan, BS
Medical Student, Albert Einstein College of Medicine, New York, New York

Contents

Part III Infrainguinal Disease

Part IV Access for Hemodialysis

16. Regulation of Angiogenesis: Mechanisms and Clinical Implications

PART I

Carotid Artery Disease

CHAPTER 1

Carotid Angioplasty and Stenting

Edward B. Diethrich, MD

Medical Director, Arizona Heart Institute and Arizona Heart Hospital,
Phoenix

Endovascular techniques have revolutionized the treatment of vascular disease, and such innovations as balloon angioplasty, stenting, and endoluminal grafting have changed treatment strategies for vascular disease considerably during the past 10 years. The management of extracranial arterial disease is not likely to be an exception, and many published results of angioplasty and stenting in the carotid artery already are encouraging.[1-17]

The Carotid and Vertebral Transluminal Angioplasty Study,[17] which included 504 patients from 24 centers in Australia, Canada, Europe, and the United States, reported equivalent safety (ie, a related stroke rate of about 10% each) and efficacy for carotid surgery and angioplasty, while indicating that angioplasty may reduce nerve injury and cardiac complications. In patients with severe coexisting carotid and coronary artery disease[12] or recurrent carotid stenosis,[16] endovascular intervention has a unique potential to provide safe and effective treatment with satisfactory mid-term patency. Patients having contralateral carotid occlusions—a subset in which endarterectomy sometimes represents a high-risk procedure—also may be treated effectively with endovascular procedures.[13]

Although the technical success rate of carotid endovascular procedures generally is excellent and continues to improve as new device designs and delivery techniques reduce the risk for procedural complications still further, the incidence of neurologic complications remains higher than we would like them to be in some series.[14] In particular, older patients (>80 years) are more likely to have complications than their younger counterparts,[15] and patients who have lesions involving the carotid bifurcation are more prone to embolization with endovascular intervention than are those with localized internal carotid stenosis.

We are moving in the direction of randomized trials that will compare carotid stenting and endarterectomy,[18,19] but many of us are concerned that it may be unethical to subject all patients to a randomization protocol that might assign them to the classic surgical procedure when there are certain subgroups of patients (eg, those who have been treated with cervical irradiation or radical neck dissection, or both) for whom angioplasty and stenting clearly seem to be preferable. The problems associated with conducting a major randomized trial are considerable.[20] Currently, fewer than 20 centers are responsible for 65% of all catheter-based carotid procedures in the United States, and an effective trial will require 40 clinical sites with trained interventionists. In addition, there is no ideal, dedicated delivery system or stent for use in carotid procedures.

Nevertheless, several trials are planned or underway. The Carotid Revascularization Endarterectomy versus Stent Trial—partially funded by the National Institutes of Health and Guidant (Indianapolis, Ind)—will evaluate the Guidant stent. No embolic protection device has yet been designated for use in this investigation. Another trial, sponsored by Cordis, (Warren, NJ) will evaluate the Smart Stent and the Angioguard protection device in a randomized study of high-risk patients. It is encouraging that these much-needed evaluations are being planned and initiated, but a great deal of time is likely to elapse before we have answers about the cost, the durability, and the relevance to clinical practice of the technology that presently is available for use in these trials. Perhaps other avenues for investigation could yield this kind of valuable information more rapidly.

GUIDELINES FOR PATIENT EVALUATION

Some carotid lesions are considerably more amenable to endovascular treatment than others, and standardizing the guidelines for patient selection for investigative procedures such as balloon angioplasty and stenting of the extracranial arteries remains somewhat problematic despite growing experience with endovascular procedures worldwide. Currently, many physicians use endovascular procedures to treat only symptomatic patients; the indications for treatment of the asymptomatic patient are more controversial. We have not definitively determined the relative efficacy and safety of endovascular procedures—particularly those involving the cervical carotid bifurcation—in comparison with carotid endarterectomy.

At the Arizona Heart Institute, either symptomatic or asymptomatic patients may be candidates for endovascular treatment of cerebrovascular disease, provided there is a clear likelihood for benefit of the endovascular procedure. We have performed more than 300 carotid endovascular procedures, the majority of which were done in asymptomatic patients who had major peripheral vascular or cardiac disease and required further intervention or surgical treatment for these problems subsequent to the correction of their carotid stenosis.

We evaluate patients for endovascular treatment according to a protocol. After an initial workup by either a cardiologist or a vascular surgeon, a neurology consultation is obtained. Noninvasive assessment with duplex imaging of the arch, vertebral, and extracranial arteries is completed, and computed tomography examination of the brain is performed. Duplex scanning has proved to be very helpful in the selection of patients for endovascular procedures. When radiolucent plaque is seen on the duplex scan, we consider the possibility that this may indicate a potentially troublesome lesion. Radiopaque (echogenic) plaque, however, often indicates a lesion that can be treated successfully using endovascular techniques. The Imaging: Carotid Angioplasty and the Risk of Stroke study is a prospective multicenter study correlating the risk of brain embolization during carotid artery stenting with plaque composition. This study is being conducted in a number of international clinical sites in an effort to formulate more definitive criteria for patient selection based on duplex evaluation.

Brain scans and magnetic resonance imaging are also used to evaluate patients as needed. Unfortunately, conventional angiographic studies often are more useful than noninvasive imaging for identifying ideal candidates for endovascular procedures; images obtained with noninvasive techniques often contain artifacts and provide less definitive resolution of the lesion and the remainder of the arterial tree. A contrast angiogram also is useful in evaluating access for the delivery of stents across torturous arch vessels.

Periprocedural stroke continues to be the most feared complication of carotid intervention, and we are hesitant to offer endovascular procedures to patients with highly complex bifurcation lesions where both duplex scanning and angiography show dense calcification and diffuse, irregular plaque. These types of lesions, which frequently extend from the common carotid artery into both the internal and external branches, often contain loose atheromatous debris. The risk of dislodging the debris during angioplasty and stenting is high, and the consequences are potentially grave. Using a number of different imaging modalities helps identify patients who may be at particular risk for perioperative cerebrovascular accidents.

We have defined 4 specific subgroups of patients in whom we believe the endovascular approach is either comparable or superior to the classic endarterectomy procedure:

1. *Patients with high internal carotid artery lesions.* Lesions that are located in the distal internal carotid artery near the base of the skull are difficult to access surgically, making them almost ideal for stenting. These lesions are far above the bifurcation, and their pathology is usually well-localized, smooth-walled, and free of loose debris. Short stents can be deployed across such lesions, keeping them completely divorced from the bifurcation area.
2. *Patients who have undergone irradiation to the cervical carotid area or have had a radical neck dissection.* Radiation to the cervical carotid area or a radical lymph node dissection may result in extensive soft tissue damage and scarring that make surgical intervention technically difficult. Stents are an ideal treatment in this setting and may be used to correct diffuse lesions along the entire course of the artery, where they trap plaque and debris against the artery wall and reduce the potential for embolic events.
3. *Patients who have had one or more previous ipsilateral carotid endarterectomy procedures.* Reoperation after endarterectomy is frequently difficult because of scarring, fibrous entrapment of adjacent cranial nerves, and cephalad extension of disease. In these patients, stent placement often is an excellent alternative. Our experience indicates lesions that occur 12 to 18 months after endarterectomy usually are caused by myointimal hyperplasia or a technical problem associated with the previous operation. These lesions generally have the appearance of a flap of plaque or a suture line that narrows the artery, and are easily corrected with stents. Lesions recurring several years after the original operation often are similar to the original atheromatous lesion, and endovascular manipulation may provoke embolization.
4. *Patients with combined or sequential lesions.* Combined procedures for dual or tandem lesions may include endarterectomy and angioplasty.[21,22] Treatment of the proximal lesion is required before or in concert with the more cephalad interven-

tion. Proximal stenosis in the innominate artery or the common carotid artery often is treated with stenting and is not particularly prone to embolization, but bifurcation lesions may require endarterectomy if loose debris is thought to be present on the basis of previous imaging studies.

TECHNIQUES FOR CAROTID ARTERY ANGIOPLASTY AND STENTING
PREPROCEDURAL CONSIDERATIONS
Most patients already take one aspirin per day, and there is no need to discontinue that regimen before the procedure. However, most interventionists now are using a dose of clopidogrel (Plavix) before stenting and are continuing this medication for 30 days after the procedure. Although there are no comparative scientific data to support this practice, it is a fairly standard approach and probably is based on the collective experience with Plavix in coronary stenting.

ANESTHESIA
Most endovascular procedures do not require the use of a general anesthetic. We prefer local anesthesia with mild sedation for percutaneous retrograde femoral interventions. Agents that allow the patient to be completely comfortable and conversant during the procedure are ideal, so that any neurologic changes may be recognized immediately. Neurologic deficits from nonembolic ischemia caused by balloon inflations are rare, and rapid deflation quickly reverses the symptoms. Balloon inflation at the carotid bifurcation more commonly causes baroreceptor stimulation with reflex bradycardia. Cardiac standstill can occur in this setting, and a brief period of sternal compression occasionally may be required. Atropine sulfate, 1 mg, administered 60 seconds before balloon expansion usually prevents this complication, but not always; therefore, careful attention must be paid to the electrocardiogram monitor during ballooning. Originally, some interventionists inserted a temporary pacing wire, but we never have considered this to be necessary.

Short-acting, rapidly reversible drugs should be used when direct access techniques are employed, so that the patient may be awakened and extubated in the endovascular suite immediately after the procedure. Although cervical block and local anesthesia have been advocated for carotid interventions, immobilizing the head and neck during the procedure is difficult, especially if the patient is not intubated and the anesthesiologist must support a mask over the patient's face. Patient movement at the time of stent deployment increases the risk of incorrect placement of the device.

ACCESS

Carotid angioplasty and stenting, like most procedures in the early development stage, require careful attention to technique. In almost every series described to date, there is a definite learning curve associated with procedural results.[1-17] Results obtained after 25 to 50 stent deployments often are more satisfactory than the experience early in a series. Deployment techniques have reached some degree of uniformity because equipment and procedures have become more specialized to accommodate the demands of carotid stenting. A detailed account of the current technical features associated with carotid stent deployment is described below.

The retrograde femoral approach is used in most endovascular procedures, although direct common carotid artery access sometimes may be indicated. A radiopaque ruler (Burkhart Roentgen, Pinellas Park, Fla) may be used for positioning relative to the target carotid artery.

Common Carotid Access

Direct percutaneous carotid access is associated with a relatively high rate of complications, and we no longer use it at our institution. The entry site into the common carotid artery can be variable distances above the clavicle, depending on the location of the lesion. Our current procedure uses a short, 2- to 3-cm incision just above the clavicle to expose the artery before inserting the needle (Fig 1). The common carotid artery is dissected free from the carotid sheath and is held with a heavy silk sling or an elastic vessel loop. This technique reduces the risk for a postprocedural hematoma and prevents stent compression that can occur using the percutaneous approach.

An 18-gauge, 2⅜-in single-wall entry needle (Cook, Inc, Bloomington, Ind) is used for the puncture. Several embolic protection devices are under development. The PercuSurge Guidewire System (PercuSurge, Inc, Sunnyvale, Calif) incorporates a distal occluding balloon and allows irrigation to carry away debris created by balloon dilation (Fig 2). Low-profile filter devices also are being studied, and early research indicates that they may markedly reduce the incidence of embolic events.[23] Several additional prototypes are being developed as well, at least one of which incorporates a filter with a 0.035-in wire—this low-profile system is particularly attractive for use during the treatment of high-grade stenotic lesions.

An angled hydrophilic guidewire, such as the Glidewire (Meditech/Boston Scientific, Watertown, Mass), is passed cephalad into the external carotid artery. Crossing the internal carotid artery is not advisable and may promote embolic complications. We use a 7F Coons dilator (Cook) to expedite the placement of a 7F, 6-cm sheath (Cordis), releasing a short bolus of contrast to confirm its position. The initial angiogram confirms the site of the lesion, but before proceeding any further, anterior-posterior and lateral cerebral angiograms are performed to establish the baseline appearance of the cerebral arteries. Roadmapping is performed using fluoroscopy, and intravenous heparin sodium (approximately 5000 units) is given to maintain the activated coagulation time above 250 seconds. Sheaths and catheters are irrigated with heparinized saline solution (10,000 units of heparin in 1000 mL of normal saline).

Angiographic visualization is used to judge the length and diameter of the lesion before any predilation. Predilation frequently is necessary before stent deployment in severely stenotic lesions, with the use of a balloon that usually is 1 or 2 sizes smaller than the stent delivery balloon, but never larger than 4 mm in diameter. The diameter and length of the lesion are assessed to determine the most appropriate stent. The most common balloon dilation catheter size is 4 mm × 2 cm, followed by stent delivery

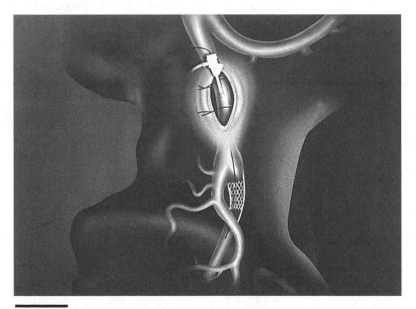

FIGURE 1.
Stylized illustration of the "mini" exposure of the common carotid artery. This technique is used when a retrograde femoral approach is not possible.

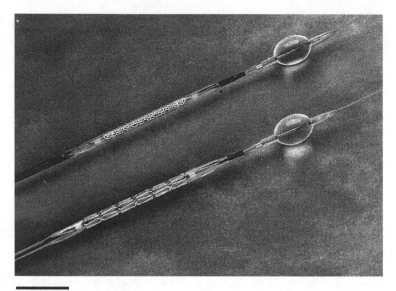

FIGURE 2.
The PercuSurge Guidewire System incorporates a distal occluding balloon and allows irrigation to carry away debris created by balloon dilation.

on a balloon of the same or the next larger size. The rigid, balloon-expandable Palmaz stent (Cordis) and the flexible, self-expanding Wallstent (Boston Scientific) are common choices; there are no stents currently approved for use in the carotid artery, but several companies are considering new prototype designs for use in this location.

The guidewire is withdrawn from the external carotid artery and is retained low in the common carotid artery to avoid any vascular trauma or arterial spasm. A smaller 0.018-in Roadrunner wire (Cook) is passed across the lesion into the internal carotid artery. Atropine sulfate, 1 mg, then is administered to prevent bradycardia and hypotension during balloon expansion.

The balloon is centered across the lesion using the roadmapping image for guidance, and a short burst of contrast is injected to document its final position. Approximately 8 to 10 atm of pressure are used for balloon expansion. If bradycardia occurs, the balloon is deflated immediately. After complete expansion, the balloon is deflated and the shaft of the angioplasty catheter is rotated to furl the balloon before it is retracted. The results of the balloon dilation are confirmed angiographically with another short burst of contrast medium. At this point, we make a final decision about the type of stent to be deployed. If a balloon-expandable stent is selected, the balloon catheter and stent are advanced into position with the stent situated between the opaque markers on the balloon. A repeat contrast injection is necessary if the patient moves. Movement or misalignment of the stent on the balloon shaft also must be avoided, even if its correct repositioning requires removal of the balloon and stent delivery catheter and starting over. Once the stent has been positioned correctly, the balloon is expanded or the self-expanding stent is released. Inflation over 3 to 5 seconds is normally adequate for the Palmaz stent.

Contrast is injected after stent deployment to confirm patency and assess proper positioning. Inadequate stent expansion may cause serious complications, such as stent occlusion and thrombus formation. Real-time intravascular ultrasound can be used to confirm proper stent deployment.[24] Finally, cerebral angiography again is performed at the conclusion of the stent deployment for comparison with the prestent image, to confirm the absence of cerebral embolization. In some cases in which emboli are visualized, neurorescue techniques—such as thrombolytic infusion—may be required, depending on the patient's clinical condition.

The results of our experience with balloon-expandable stents have been excellent. Although stent deformity has been reported, we have not observed it since we started using our "mini" exposure technique instead of direct carotid puncture. Long-term patency without intimal hyperplasia has encouraged us to continue using these types of stents (Fig 3). However, in spite of our very encouraging results with Palmaz stents, most of our current stenting procedures are accomplished with self-expanding stents, many of which are constructed with a nitinol framework.

Once the procedure is complete, the incision is closed and anesthesia may be discontinued. Blood pressure should be monitored closely because uncontrolled hypertension may result in significant hematoma formation. The patient should be awakened and assessed for any neurologic deficits before transfer to the intensive care unit. Within the first hour after transfer, we perform a duplex scan of the treatment site.

Femoral Access

Retrograde femoral access is the approach that is used most frequently for endovascular intervention. Both iliac arteries are evaluated to determine the side with the less tortuous and stenotic artery. Atherosclerotic occlusion of the abdominal aorta or the iliac or femoral vessels precludes retrograde femoral access, and either a direct approach or transbrachial catheterization must be used in

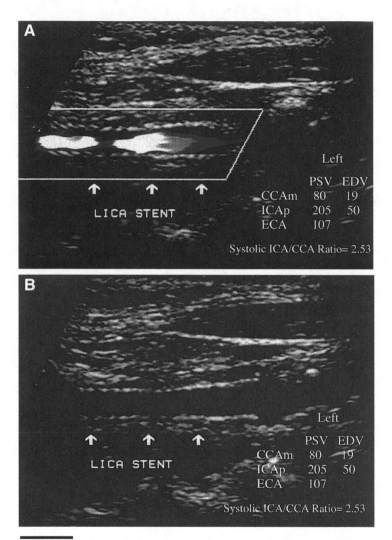

FIGURE 3.
Color-flow duplex **(A)** and gray-scale ultrasound scans **(B)** in a patient who had a Palmaz 204 stent (arrows) placed for the treatment of symptomatic internal carotid artery stenosis 5 years earlier. Note the excellent flow and the absence of either stent deformity or myointimal hyperplasia. *Abbreviations*: *LICA*, left internal carotid artery; *ICA*, internal carotid artery; *CCA*, common carotid artery; *ECA*, external carotid artery; *CCAm*, common carotid artery mean; *ICA*, internal carotid artery peak; *PSV*, peak systolic velocity; *EDV*, end diastolic volume.

these cases. An 18-gauge, 2 ⅜-in needle is inserted in the common femoral artery and followed by a 0.035-in guidewire (Glidewire, Medi-tech/Boston Scientific) and a 7F or 9F sheath (Cordis). Intravenous heparin (approximately 5000 units) is administered, and a 260-cm, 0.035-in angled hydrophilic guidewire (Medi-tech) is passed into the aortic arch. A JB2 catheter (Cook), or another catheter of similar design, is passed into the high ascending aorta, and the wire is withdrawn to expose the angle of the JB2 catheter. The catheter then is withdrawn slowly to selectively engage either the brachiocephalic trunk or the origin of the left common carotid artery.

After the angled guidewire has been passed into the appropriate common carotid artery, the JB2 catheter is advanced over it to the mid-level of the carotid artery. The angled guidewire then is introduced into the external carotid artery, followed by the JB2 catheter. The guidewire is removed and replaced with a 260-cm Super Stiff Amplatz wire (Cook), which is passed into the external carotid artery. The JB2 catheter is removed, and the fluoroscope is panned in the anterior-posterior position from the cervical carotid artery across the arch to allow assessment of the angle and origin of the great vessels containing the Amplatz wire. The operator should observe the angle of the vessels carefully; an angle that is too acute at the carotid or innominate artery junction may make angioplasty and stent deployment difficult or impossible. Conversion to the open approach may be appropriate when vessel angles are too acute.

A flexible delivery catheter, such as the Flexor catheter (Cook), is inserted into the mid-carotid position, the Amplatz wire is removed, and a 0.014-in Roadrunner wire is passed across the lesion in the internal carotid artery. Contrast is injected for cerebral visualization in 2 views and followed by roadmapping; the dimensions of the artery and the nature and length of the lesion are also determined. In some cases, a stent can be deployed without ballooning. When ballooning is required, a small balloon (4 mm × 2 cm) with a 120-cm shaft length is selected and passed to the lesion. After atropine has been administered, the balloon is inflated for a few seconds at 8 to 10 atm. At this point in the procedure, a small bolus of contrast medium is injected to assess the angioplasty result.

Once a stent has been selected and passed to the lesion, a second contrast bolus is injected to confirm proper location. The Palmaz stent is deployed using a 3- to 5-second balloon inflation, or the self-expanding Wallstent is released quickly into the vessel.

If there is any question regarding proper deployment, an intravascular ultrasound study is performed. When deployment is adequate, a final control angiogram that includes the intracranial circulation is performed. If deployment has been inadequate, additional dilation of the stent with a larger balloon is necessary. In most cases in which a self-expanding stent is used, postdeployment balloon dilation is required near the midpoint of the lesion.

After dilation, the guiding catheter is withdrawn into the descending thoracic aorta, and a short 9F sheath is substituted in the groin. The patient is then transferred to the intensive care unit for observation and duplex scanning. The groin sheath is removed when the activated coagulation time returns to normal. Pseudoaneurysm and arteriovenous fistula are potential complications of femoral access, but the most common complication is a groin hematoma, which may be prevented by careful sheath removal and attention to the patient's coagulation status.

DISCUSSION

From the description above, it is clear that many of the technical features of carotid angioplasty and stenting have evolved enough that anecdotal results in carefully selected patients are very similar to those seen with carotid endarterectomy. There is considerable sentiment to compare endovascular procedures and endarterectomy in a formal, randomized trial as proposed by the The Carotid Revascularization Endarterectomy versus Stent Trial investigators.

It already appears that patients who leave the hospital without a periprocedural complication of carotid stenting are not likely to have serious neurologic events—indeed, the risk of such an event after discharge seems to be comparable to the same risk after carotid endarterectomy. More problematic is the risk of stroke within the first 24 hours after the carotid endovascular procedure, and a number of embolic protection devices are currently being evaluated in an effort to prevent these complications. The PercuSurge and Angioguard devices have been tested most extensively, but a novel device with a 0.035-in wire configuration (Fig 4) also is being tested by Embolic Protection, Inc (San Carlos, Calif). We are hopeful that other devices will be designed to support stenting in the carotid bifurcation and in other locations where complex lesions otherwise would increase the risk of periprocedural stroke.

At present, carotid angioplasty and stenting must be considered an investigational procedure despite its early success in carefully selected patient populations. In fact, relatively few physicians favor the use of endovascular procedures for the majority of carotid interventions. A group of experienced authorities from several disciplines was assembled to address the controversies surrounding carotid angioplasty and stenting at the Consensus Conference on Endovascular Therapies (New York, NY, September 18-21, 1999). The results of this consensus panel will be published but, in the meantime, it is useful to consider the various viewpoints of these interventional cardiologists, radiologists, and vascular surgeons.

When presented with the question regarding whether carotid angioplasty and stenting should become the standard of care before data from a randomized trial are available, the majority of physicians on the panel responded that it should not. Nevertheless, many panel members agreed that endovascular procedures cur-

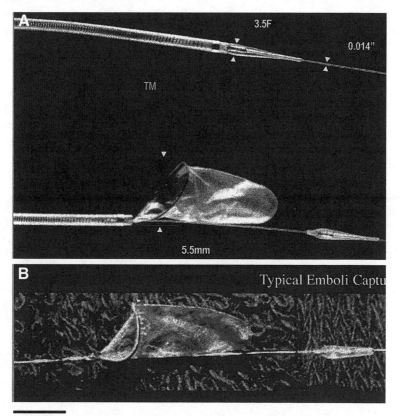

FIGURE 4.
A, The device that has been designed by Embolic Protection, Inc, to prevent distal embolization during carotid stenting procedures. **B,** Typical embolic debris captured by this device.

rently are justified for the treatment of high-risk, symptomatic patients or those with high internal carotid artery lesions, contralateral internal carotid artery occlusions, ipsilateral recurrent stenosis, or a history of cervical irradiation or radical neck dissection. Although panelists agreed that patients who are considered to be unfit for surgery represent candidates for endovascular intervention, the guidelines for determining "fitness" were a topic of considerable debate. As defined by the panel, carotid endovascular procedures are contraindicated for patients in whom access was severely limited or who had sustained a recent cerebrovascular accident. Carotid stenting also was thought to be contraindicated in patients with complex lesions, or lesions that either contained intraluminal thrombus or were extensively calcified.

Panel members were evenly divided on the question of whether institutions should be required to obtain an Investigational Device Exemption from the Food and Drug Administration before offering carotid endovascular procedures. Currently, the majority of institutions in which these procedures are performed have not obtained an Investigational Device Exemption.

Although periprocedural stroke remains the most serious complication of carotid stenting, the prevailing opinion of the panel members was that the procedure could be performed without the use of an embolic protection device. Perhaps this is not surprising, given that the devices are not currently available to most centers. All panelists agreed, however, that these devices should be used routinely as soon as they are more widely distributed.

Panelists would like more variety in equipment choices for carotid endovascular procedures, and they encouraged the design of new devices for specific use above the aortic arch. Indeed, there is concern that equipment has not evolved quickly enough to keep pace with advances in technique. In our experience, changes in patient selection and technique have dramatically reduced the incidence of complications. An analysis of results in a current series of 179 patients indicates a procedural success rate of 96% and a 3.6% rate of neurologic complications. The overall rate of death and neurologic complications decreased from 10.9% in our initial series,[4] to 6.2% in the current series, despite the fact that a subset of our most recent patients had combined lesions at the level of the carotid bifurcation, which are difficult to treat.

CONCLUSION

Carotid angioplasty and stenting remain controversial, and many physicians maintain their preference for endarterectomy, despite significant advancements in endovascular techniques and improvements in procedural success rates. Many of us continue to believe that carotid endovascular procedures are safe and effective in treating certain types of lesions. Patient selection is extremely important in the success of these procedures, and the planning of randomized trials should reflect the state of our current knowledge regarding procedural indications and contraindications. Although endovascular intervention is not likely to obviate the need for endarterectomy, it seems certain to have an important place in the treatment of carotid vascular disease.

REFERENCES

1. Kachel R, Basche S, Heerklotz I, et al: Percutaneous transluminal angioplasty of supra-aortic arteries, especially the internal carotid artery. *Neuroradiology* 33:191-194, 1991.
2. Kachel R: Results of balloon angioplasty in the carotid arteries. *J Endovasc Surg* 3:22-30, 1996.
3. Theron J: Angioplastie carotidienne protegee et stents carotidiens. *J Mal Vasc* 21:113S-122S, 1996.
4. Diethrich EB, Ndiaye M, Reid DB: Stenting in the carotid artery: Initial experience in 110 patients. *J Endovasc Surg* 3:42-62, 1996.
5. Wholey MH, Wholey M, Jarmolowski CR, et al: Endovascular stents for carotid artery occlusive disease. *J Endovasc Surg* 4:326-338, 1997.
6. Teitlebaum GP, Lefkowitz MA, Giannotta SL: Carotid angioplasty and stenting in high-risk patients. *Surg Neurol* 50:300-311, 1998.
7. Wholey MH, Wholey M, Bergeron P, et al: Current global status of carotid artery stent placement. *Cathet Cardiovasc Diagn* 44:1-6, 1998.
8. Jordan WD Jr, Voellinger DC, Doblar DD, et al: Microemboli detected by transcranial Doppler monitoring in patients during carotid angioplasty versus carotid endarterectomy. *Cardiovasc Surg* 7:33-38, 1999.
9. Jordan WD Jr, Schroeder PT, Fisher WS, et al: A comparison of angioplasty with stenting versus endarterectomy for the treatment of carotid artery stenosis. *Ann Vasc Surg* 11:2-8, 1997.
10. Jordan WD Jr, Roye GD, Fisher WS III, et al: A cost comparison of balloon angioplasty and stenting versus endarterectomy for the treatment of carotid artery stenosis. *J Vasc Surg* 27:16-22, 1998.
11. National Stroke Association: Current status of carotid stenting. *Stroke Clin Update* IX:1-4, 1999.
12. Al-Mubarak N, Roubin GS, Liu MW, et al: Early results of percutaneous intervention for severe coexisting carotid and coronary artery disease. *Am J Cardiol* 84:600-602, 1999.
13. Mericle RA, Kim SH, Lanzino G, et al: Carotid artery angioplasty and use of stents in high-risk patients with contralateral occlusions. *J Neurosurg* 90:1031-1036, 1999.
14. Leisch F, Kershner K, Hofman R, et al: Carotid stenting: Acute results and complications. *Z Kardiol* 88:661-668, 1999.

15. Chastain HD II, Gomez CR, Iyer S, et al: Influence of age upon complications of carotid artery stenting. *J Endovasc Surg* 3:217-222, 1999.
16. Lanzino G, Mericle RA, Lopes DK, et al: Percutaneous transluminal angioplasty and stent placement for recurrent carotid artery stenosis. *J Neurosurg* 90:688-694, 1999.
17. Brown MM: Vascular Surgical Society of Great Britain and Ireland: Results of the Carotid and Vertebral Artery Transluminal Angioplasty Study. *Br J Surg* 86:710-711, 1999.
18. Hobson RW II, Brott T, Ferguson R, et al: CREST: Carotid Revascularization Endarterectomy versus Stent Trial. *Cardiovasc Surg* 5:457-458, 1997.
19. Diethrich EB: Carotid angioplasty and stenting. Will they match the gold standard? *Tex Heart Inst J* 25:1-9, 1998.
20. Wholey MH: Randomizing carotid endarterectomy to carotid stenting? *J Endovasc Surg* 6:127-129, 1999.
21. Levien LJ, Benn CA, Veller MG, et al: Retrograde balloon angioplasty of brachiocephalic or common carotid artery stenoses at the time of carotid endarterectomy. *Eur J Vasc Endovasc Surg* 15:521-527, 1998.
22. Sidhu PS, Morgan MB, Walters HL, et al: Technical report: Combined carotid bifurcation endarterectomy and intraoperative transluminal angioplasty of a proximal common carotid artery stenosis: An alternative to extrathoracic bypass. *Clin Radiol* 53:444-447, 1998.
23. Ohki T, Roubin GS, Veith FJ, et al: Efficacy of filter device in the prevention of embolic events during carotid angioplasty and stenting: An ex vivo analysis. *J Vasc Surg* 30:1034-1044, 1999.
24. Reid DB, Diethrich EB, Marx P, et al: Intravascular ultrasound assessment in carotid interventions. *J Endovasc Surg* 3:203-210, 1996.

CHAPTER 2

Carotid Angioplasty and Stenting: A Personal Perspective

Kenneth Ouriel, MD
Chairman, Department of Vascular Surgery, The Cleveland Clinic Foundation, Cleveland, Ohio

Jay S. Yadav, MD
Associate Professor of Medicine, Ohio State University, Cleveland; Director, Carotid Interventions, The Cleveland Clinic Foundation, Cleveland, Ohio

No peripheral vascular surgical procedure has been subjected to such extreme scrutiny as carotid endarterectomy. Since the first carotid repair for symptomatic disease was conducted by the Argentine authors Carrea et al[1] in 1951, the procedure has been investigated with a wide array of well-designed and well-executed clinical trials. In fact, a multicenter trial comparing the surgical and medical management of carotid disease was organized within a decade of Carrea's report, and the results of a randomized comparison of more than 1200 patients appeared in a series of publications in the late 1960s and early 1970s. The benefit of surgical over medical management of carotid disease was well elucidated by W. S. Fields[2] more than 3 decades ago, when he proclaimed:

> A patient who has localized disease in the cervical carotid arteries, either unilateral or bilateral, with stenosis of greater than 50%, tends to have fewer transient and recurrent attacks of neurological deficit during follow-up after surgery.

Despite the findings of this large trial, enthusiasm for carotid repair waned during the following decade. In the late 1980s, however, a series of clinical trials were instituted, including the North American Symptomatic Carotid Endarterectomy Trial (NASCET),[3] the European Carotid Surgery Trial (ECST), and the Asymptomatic

Carotid Artery Surgery Trial (ACAS). In spite of questions regarding the efficacy of the procedure at the commencement of every trial, the final data exonerated carotid endarterectomy each time.

With the demonstration of the efficacy of coronary angioplasty and stenting, investigators became interested in a percutaneous treatment for carotid disease. The large number of patients with suitable carotid lesions sparked interest on the part of industry, and, despite a national "noncoverage" policy for carotid angioplasty by the Health Care Financing Administration (HCFA), carotid stenting became one of the most widely discussed and hotly debated topics of the late 1990s. Interventional cardiologists, well versed in percutaneous angioplasty and with nothing to lose and much to gain, were quick to embrace the new technology. Vascular surgeons, by contrast, viewed carotid angioplasty as a rather crude and yet unproved threat to the meticulous procedure of carotid endarterectomy, one of the mainstays of contemporary peripheral vascular surgical practice. With neurologists and neurosurgeons in the middle, a conflict ensued, the resolution of which could only be achieved through the completion of well-controlled comparisons of the 2 treatment modalities.

LIMITATIONS OF STANDARD THERAPY FOR CAROTID DISEASE

Carotid endarterectomy is a well-proved intervention for carotid disease. The results of numerous clinical trials have documented its safety and efficacy so well that it remains the standard of care for patients with severely stenotic extracranial lesions, whether the patient is symptomatic or not. Nevertheless, the excellent results achieved with the procedure appear to be dependent on the baseline medical status of the patient. Not unexpectedly, relatively healthy patients do very well with open surgical repair of carotid lesions. The treatment of medically compromised patients, however, is associated with a much greater risk of complications, as illustrated in a review of more than 3000 patients undergoing carotid endarterectomy at the Cleveland Clinic Foundation between 1988 and 1998. In this analysis of a consecutive series of patients, the risk of the composite end point of stroke, myocardial infarction, or death was satisfactory in patients who did not manifest 1 of 5 classes of baseline comorbidity (Table 1). The risk of perioperative morbidity and mortality was substantial, however, when patients had one or more baseline comorbid conditions (Fig 1). Specifically, the risk of perioperative death was elevated by a factor of more than 5, stroke or myocardial infarction each by a factor of 2, and the composite end point of death, stroke, or myocardial infarction by a factor of almost 3.

TABLE 1.
Rate of Perioperative Complications in High- and Low-risk Patients Undergoing Carotid Endarterectomy at the Cleveland Clinic[5]

Risk Group	Indication	Total Pts	% Total	D/S/MI*	%	Death	%	Stroke	%	MI	%
High risk	Asymp	436	73.4	30	6.9	16	3.7	14	3.2	5	1.1
	TIA	107	18.0	9	8.4	6	5.6	4	3.7	3	2.8
	Stroke	51	8.6	5	9.8	4	7.8	3	5.9	2	3.9
	Total	594	19.4	44	7.4	26	4.4	21	3.5	10	1.7
Low risk	Asymp	1542	62.5	36	2.3	3	0.2	18	1.2	18	1.2
	TIA	635	25.7	19	3.0	2	0.3	16	2.5	3	0.5
	Stroke	290	11.8	16	5.5	3	1.0	8	2.8	6	2.1
	Total	2467	80.6	71	2.9	8	0.3	42	1.7	27	1.1
All	Asymp	1978	64.6	66	3.3	19	1.0	32	1.6	23	1.2
	TIA	742	24.2	28	3.8	8	1.1	20	2.7	6	0.8
	Stroke	341	11.1	21	6.2	7	2.1	11	3.2	8	2.3
	Total	3061	100.0	115	3.8	34	1.1	63	2.1	37	1.2

*D/S/MI signifies the rate of the composite end point death, stroke, or myocardial infarction.
Abbreviations: TIA, Transient ischemic attack; *Asymp*, asymptomatic.

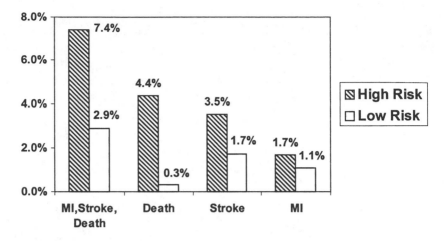

FIGURE 1.
The risk of stroke, myocardial infarction *(MI)*, or death, as a composite
end point and separately, in 3061 high- and low-risk patients undergoing
carotid endarterectomy at the Cleveland Clinic.[5]

The interpretation of the Cleveland Clinic data is that, in most
cases, carotid endarterectomy is a procedure with an extremely
low rate of complications. In studies that specifically exclude
high-risk patients from eligibility, for example, the NASCET and
ACAS trials, the rate of periprocedural complications can be
expected to be extremely low. When casually reviewing these trials, it would be a grave error to assume that the results of carotid
endarterectomy presented herein are similar to those in unselected
patients undergoing carotid repair at the "grass roots" level. On the
contrary, data exist suggesting that the results of the trials cannot
even be generalized to patients undergoing endarterectomy at the
hospitals that participated in the studies. In a study of 113,000
Medicare patients who underwent carotid endarterectomy during
patient acquisition for the NASCET and ACAS trials (1992–1993),
Wennberg et al[4] noted that the perioperative mortality rate was
1.4% in hospitals participating in the trials and 1.7% in hospitals
that did not participate in the trials. The rate of perioperative
death rose to 2.5% in low-volume nontrial hospitals where fewer
than 7 carotid endarterectomies were performed yearly. These relatively high complication rates are in direct contrast to the much
lower mortality rates observed in the patients entered into the trials (0.1% in ACAS and 0.6% in NASCET). These findings suggest
that eligibility criteria were sufficiently strict that patients in the
NASCET and ACAS trials represented a small subset of the total

population of patients undergoing carotid endarterectomy, comprising a subgroup with the lowest frequency of baseline comorbid conditions and, likely, the lowest rate of perioperative adverse events.

The data from the Cleveland Clinic registry[5] offer an explanation for Wennberg's findings. Patients in the multicenter trials of carotid endarterectomy were similar to the low-risk group of patients undergoing carotid repair at the Cleveland Clinic. In fact, the mortality rate of 0.2% in more than 1500 "low-risk" asymptomatic patients treated with carotid endarterectomy is remarkably similar to the ACAS mortality rate of 0.1%. Similarly, the mortality rate was 0.5% in 925 symptomatic patients undergoing carotid endarterectomy at the Cleveland Clinic, almost identical to the 0.6% mortality rate observed in the NASCET trial.

These observations have implications in the design of trials aimed at assessing carotid stenting procedures. Periprocedural morbidity is likely to be highest during the relatively early evolution of stent design and stenting treatment paradigms. At a time when the safety and efficacy of carotid stenting remains unproved, investigations seem most appropriately undertaken in the population of patients with less ideal outcomes after the standard therapy of carotid endarterectomy. To evaluate carotid stenting versus endarterectomy in a subgroup known for its low rate of perioperative morbidity jeopardizes successfully demonstrating equivalence between stenting and endarterectomy, resulting in the premature abandonment of the new technology. It is the authors' opinion that the true benefit of carotid stenting is in the reduction of periprocedural myocardial infarction and death—events that are correlated with the invasiveness of the intervention. Given this hypothesis, the probability of demonstrating equivalence between carotid stenting and carotid endarterectomy will be less likely in a patient population with a low rate of perioperative complications, especially if stenting proves to be associated with a slightly higher rate of perioperative stroke.

In addition to baseline comorbidities, a variety of anatomical features are also associated with poorer outcome. These include such variables as contralateral carotid occlusion,[3] recurrent carotid lesions,[6] and a history of radiation therapy to the neck.[7] These issues may be important in determining the outcome with open carotid procedures, with regard to perioperative stroke, myocardial infarction, and death, as well as softer end points such as wound complications and cranial nerve injury. These anatomical features should also be taken into account in the differentiation between high- and low-risk patients. Complications that are associated with the invasive nature of open surgery would be likely to occur at a lower frequency in the stented subgroup. As such, both clinical and anatomical baseline variables should be addressed when delineating a high-risk patient population suitable for an initial investigation of endarterectomy versus stenting.

CATEGORIES OF DISEASE APPROPRIATE FOR CAROTID STENTING

The etiology of carotid bifurcation disease can be categorized into atherosclerotic and nonatherosclerotic processes, the former seen much more frequently than the latter in clinical practice. The nonatherosclerotic causes of carotid bifurcation disease may be further subdivided into the inflammatory problems such as Takaysu arteritis, postendarterectomy intimal hyperplasia, and carotid stenosis caused by spontaneous dissections. It is attractive to hypothesize that the short-term results of carotid stenting would be best in patients with nonatherosclerotic disease, because the lesions are, by and large, smooth. As such, the potential for embolization is theoretically lower than that associated with complex atherosclerotic lesions. Many of these disease entities produce long, tapered carotid lesions, rendering them exceedingly difficult to treat with any modality. In addition, hypercoagulable problems may occur in association with some of the nonatherosclerotic etiologies, raising the risk of early postprocedural thrombosis. Clearly, the treatment of patients with the more esoteric causes of carotid stenosis is complicated, based on little more than anecdotal experience, and, as such, should involve consultative input from a broad spectrum of specialists including rheumatologists, hematologists, and vascular medicine practitioners.

In patients with atherosclerotic disease, the risk of carotid stenting is correlated with the extent of the atherosclerotic process. Patients with diffuse disease involving the aortic arch and common carotid vessels should be viewed with caution, as should patients with significant intracranial disease. The heavily calcified, tortuous vessel is one fraught with difficulty, and the use of alternate treatment modalities should be strongly considered.

TECHNIQUE OF CAROTID STENTING

Anecdotal evidence exists to suggest that the glycoprotein IIb/IIIa platelet antagonists may be of benefit in patients undergoing the placement of a carotid stent. The use of agents such as abciximab (ReoPro, Centocor, Malvern, Pa), eptifibatide (Integrilin, Cor Therapeutics, La Jolla, Calif), and tirofiban (Aggrastat, Merck, West

Point, Pa) makes theoretical sense, given the presumed increase in thrombogenicity of the stented luminal surface. Abciximab is a large Fc fragment with activity against not only the platelet glycoprotein IIb/IIIa receptor, but also the MAC_1 and the $\alpha_v\beta_3$ receptor. It has the potential to block leukocyte chemotaxis and smooth muscle cell migration—two processes that are intimately involved in restenosis. By contrast, the small molecules eptifibatide and tirofiban possess specific activity against the glycoprotein receptors alone, limiting action to platelet-mediated events such as immediate stent thrombosis. Empirical and somewhat circumstantial evidence from the coronary literature supports this contention. In stented diabetic patients treated with abciximab, the need for repeat revascularization, a surrogate end point for restenosis, was lower than in those not receiving the agent. No such preventive effect was noted in trials of the small molecules eptifibatide and tirofiban, suggesting that their actions are limited to the platelet. In view of these observations, we have used abciximab in a 0.25 mg/kg bolus loading dose followed by a 0.125 µg/kg per minute infusion for 12 hours after the procedure. The use of eptifibatide or tirofiban has theoretical advantages when an open surgical procedure such as coronary artery bypass is anticipated to be necessary within a few days of carotid stenting, given the longer half-life of abciximab. In practice, abciximab is readily and instantaneously reversible with platelet transfusions, whereas the small molecules are not. In this regard, protracted platelet dysfunction despite platelet transfusion has been, in our experience, almost universally the result of clopidogrel and aspirin rather than the glycoprotein IIb/IIIa inhibitors.

The procedure of carotid stenting commences with a high-quality diagnostic arteriographic study of the cerebrovasculature. Failure to detect a carotid bifurcation lesion of the severity suggested by a previous duplex scan should prompt one to obtain as many oblique projections as necessary, since contemporary, well-performed duplex studies may be more sensitive than single or dual-projection contrast arteriography. One should be certain to obtain adequate views of the intracranial vasculature, to document any postprocedural changes resulting from iatrogenic embolization.

After diagnostic arteriography, the patient is heparinized and a 0.035-in Glide wire is advanced through the diagnostic catheter into the external carotid artery. The diagnostic catheter is advanced over the wire and into the external carotid vessel, thereafter exchanging the Glide wire for a 0.035-in super-stiff guidewire. The diagnostic catheter is exchanged for a 9F guide catheter, which is placed at the level of the mid–common carotid artery. Once the guiding catheter has been threaded to a level just below the carotid lesion, the lesion is crossed with a fine (eg, 0.014 in) guidewire. Alternatively, an embolic protection device may be used at this point, if available. Various devices can function as the guidewire for subsequent angioplasty and stenting; for example, AngioGuard, (Cordis, Miami, Fla) and NeuroShield (MedNova, Galway, Ireland), both of which use distal internal carotid artery filters that maintain antegrade flow during the procedure. Other devices use proximal or distal occluding balloons (PercuSurge and ArteriA) to arrest antegrade blood flow and allow aspiration of debris through a proximal guide catheter or sheath.

Once the lesion has been crossed with a wire, the lesion is "predilated" with a 3- or 4-mm balloon. Next, a self-expanding stent of an appropriate diameter and length is positioned across the lesion, and the sheath is retracted to allow deployment. "Postdilation" with an appropriate-sized balloon (usually 5-7 mm) is usually necessary, followed by completion arteriography with extracranial and intracranial views. After a satisfactory clinical and arteriographic result has been achieved (Fig 2), the sheath is removed and the femoral access site is sealed with a closure device such as the Perclose system (Perclose, Redwood City, Calif) to limit the risk of bleeding secondary to platelet inhibition.

STRATEGY FOR APPROVAL OF DEVICES BY THE US FOOD AND DRUG ADMINISTRATION (FDA)

The approval of medical devices by the FDA is covered within the Federal Code of Regulations. Devices that were in use before 1976 are excluded from these regulations and, in fact, new devices must be shown to be superior to or at least not inferior to a pre1976 device. In some cases, the FDA has determined that a "510(k)" pathway is appropriate for approval, usually when the device is deemed "non-critical." In these scenarios, the device is merely shown to be equivalent to a pre1976 device with clinical or even nonclinical data. Once data have been submitted, the FDA has 60 days in which to notify the marketer whether the device may be sold or, alternatively, that the data submitted are inadequate to justify similarity to the comparator device and additional information is necessary. Biliary stents are a prime example of devices where a 510(k) pathway was acceptable. Once approved for the biliary indication, the same devices were used "off-label" in the treatment of iliac or renal disease.

By contrast, dedicated carotid stents, like coronary stents, must follow the "premarket approval" (PMA) pathway. A PMA strategy

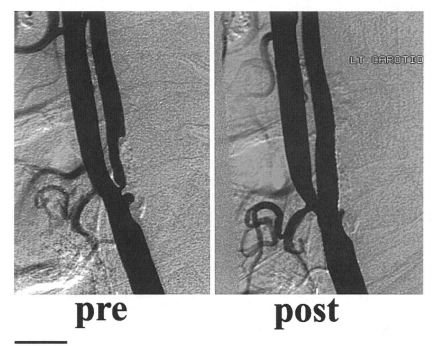

pre   post

FIGURE 2.
Before and after arteriographic views of the carotid artery treated with angioplasty and stenting.

is much more complex than the 510(k) pathway. Clinical studies are necessary, usually directed at a comparison between the new device and standard treatment. In the case of carotid stents, standard therapy is carotid endarterectomy. The carotid revascularization endarterectomy versus stent and study of angioplasty with distal protection in patients at high risk for endarterectomy clinical trials have chosen to randomly assign patients to carotid stenting or carotid endarterectomy, and at least the latter trial was designed to gain approval for marketing of the carotid stent and adjuvants (delivery system and emboli protection device). Approval of a carotid stent for marketing will be dependent on the successful completion of a trial that uses a clinically relevant primary end point (eg, stroke, death, or the composite end point of stroke, myocardial infarction, or death) to demonstrate one of the following:

1. Superiority of the device over open carotid repair, with an α probability (type I error) of 5% or less.

2. Noninferiority of the device in comparison with open repair, with an α probability of 5% or less (95% certainty) that outcome in the stented patients is not more than a predetermined percentage (the "delta") worse than standard therapy. The appropriate level for the delta value remains a topic of discussion.

REIMBURSEMENT FOR CAROTID ANGIOPLASTY AND STENTING

The HCFA determined that carotid angioplasty should not be reimbursable to Medicare beneficiaries because of a lack of data documenting clinical benefit. As such, in 1988 HCFA issued a "noncoverage" policy for carotid angioplasty, specifically excluding reimbursement for angioplasty of the cerebrovasculature. More than a dozen years have passed since the issuance of this policy, and many HCFA teams have come and gone. Thus, it is not surprising that the original intent of the policy is ill-defined, and we are left to guess whether its authors meant to exclude carotid stenting or merely balloon angioplasty of the carotid vessels. Nevertheless, once a noncoverage policy has been issued, neither the casual use of the technique nor careful clinical investigatory procedures are reimbursable to the physician in the form of Medicare Part B professional fees or to the hospital by way of Medicare Part A remuneration. This dilemma is associated with a "catch-22" phenomenon whereby percutaneous carotid intervention cannot be reimbursed because of a lack of data documenting medical necessity (benefit), yet scientific studies aimed at evaluation of efficacy cannot be performed unless the treating physician and the hospital are willing to provide services for study patients on a pro bono basis, or the manufacturer is willing to reimburse costs to the health care providers. At present, both HCFA and the clinical trialists are working to address this problem. It is hoped that a strategy for reimbursement of study patients will be devised, without opening up the floodgates to the willy-nilly performance of carotid stenting at large.

CONCLUSION

Although it may be unrealistic to assume that the results of carotid stenting will attain clinical equipoise with endarterectomy in all patient subgroups, it seems reasonable to predict that this potentially less invasive procedure will result in a lower complication rate in medically compromised, "high-risk" patients. If "noninferiority" of carotid stenting cannot be demonstrated in this group of patients with less ideal outcomes after carotid endarterectomy, it is unlikely that stenting can compete successfully with endarterectomy in a lower risk group. These considerations argue for limiting the initial evaluation of stenting to a select subset of the population with carotid disease; a subset in whom standard therapy has been associated with a high rate of complications on the basis of significant baseline medical comorbidities.

REFERENCES

1. Carrea R, Molins M, Murphy G: Surgical treatment of spontaneous thrombosis of the internal carotid artery in the neck. Carotid-carotideal anastomosis. Report of a case. *Acta Neurol Latinoamer* 1:17, 1955.
2. Fields WS, Maslenikov V, Meyer JS, et al: Joint study of extracranial arterial occlusion: V. Progress report of prognosis following surgery or nonsurgical treatment for transient cerebral ischemic attacks and cervical carotid artery lesions. *JAMA* 211:1993-2003, 1970.
3. Barnett HJ, Taylor DW, Eliasziw M, et al: Benefit of carotid endarterectomy in patients with symptomatic moderate or severe stenosis. North American Symptomatic Carotid Endarterectomy Trial Collaborators. *N Engl J Med* 339:1415-1425, 1998.
4. Wennberg DE, Lucas FL, Birkmeyer JD, et al: Variation in carotid endarterectomy mortality in the Medicare population: Trial hospitals, volume, and patient characteristics. *JAMA* 279:1278-1281, 1998.
5. Ouriel K, Hertzer NR, Beven EG, et al: Pre-procedural risk stratification: Identifying an appropriate group in whom to study the role of carotid stenting. *Circulation* 100:I-67, 1999.
6. Rockman CB, Riles TS, Landis R, et al: Redo carotid surgery: An analysis of materials and configurations used in carotid reoperations and their influence on perioperative stroke and subsequent recurrent stenosis. *J Vasc Surg* 29:72-80, 1999.
7. Kashyap VS, Moore WS, Quinones-Baldrich WJ: Carotid artery repair for radiation-associated atherosclerosis is a safe and durable procedure. *J Vasc Surg* 29:90-96, 1999.

PART II

Aortic Disease

C HAPTER 3

Pararenal Aortic Aneurysms: The Future of Open Repair

Louis M. Messina, MD
Professor of Surgery, Chief, Division of Vascular Surgery, University of California, San Francisco

Linda Reilly, MD
Professor of Surgery, University of California, San Francisco

Recent developments in stent-graft technology have had a dramatic impact on the management of abdominal aortic aneurysms (AAAs). Currently, endovascular repair is feasible in approximately 60% of all infrarenal AAAs.[1] The most important factor in determining the feasibility of endovascular repair is the anatomy of the proximal aortic implantation site. The most common contraindication to the deployment of an endovascular stent-graft device for AAA repair is the lack of an adequate proximal implantation site because of aneurysmal degeneration of the pararenal aorta.

One implication of the widespread use of stent-grafts for the repair of AAAs is that an increasing proportion of patients undergoing standard open repair will have juxtarenal aneurysms requiring suprarenal crossclamp, suprarenal aneurysms requiring renal artery reconstruction, or juxtarenal aneurysms with associated renal artery occlusive disease requiring treatment. Pararenal aortic aneurysm repair is characterized by more extensive mobilization of the viscera to provide extended proximal exposure of the aorta, a more proximal level of aortic crossclamping, and an obligatory period of renal ischemia. As a result of these factors, pararenal aortic aneurysm repair is associated with a higher risk of death or complications than is infrarenal aortic repair because of its greater physiologic and cardiac stresses, as well as an increased risk of loss of renal function caused by the obligatory period of renal ischemia.

Although there have been many large referral-based[2] and population-based[3-6] studies that established the outcome of standard open operative repair of infrarenal aortic aneurysms, there are few data regarding the outcome of treatment of pararenal aortic aneurysms. Ernst[2] pooled data from several referral-based studies and reported an overall mortality rate of 3.5% (range, 1.5%-5.1%) for routine repair of nonruptured infrarenal AAA. During the last 8 years at the University of California, San Francisco (UCSF), the mortality rate of infrarenal aortic aneurysms in our referral population is 3.1%. Mortality rates for AAA repair reported from population-based studies are higher, ranging from 4.6% to 7.6%. For example, Katz et al[3] reported a mortality rate of 7.5% for AAA repair in Michigan from 1980 to 1990, remarkably similar to the results reported in a recent review of statewide aneurysm repair from California, which cited a mortality rate of 7.6%.[4] Johnston and Scobie[6] reported a mortality rate of 4.8% in their Canadian population-based study, and finally, the Veterans Affairs Aneurysm Detection and Management study reported a perioperative mortality rate of 4.9%.[5]

There are relatively few studies reporting the results of pararenal aortic aneurysm repair, and all of these published studies are referral-based. The first published series, by Crawford et al,[7] reported a mortality rate of 7.9%, largely attributed to the complications of acute postoperative renal failure. In an earlier series from UCSF[8] involving 77 patients, a mortality rate of 1.3% was reported. Since that report, 7 additional series have been published, with mortality rates varying from 0% to 10%.[9-15] These series are weighted heavily toward patients with juxtarenal aneurysms and include only a few patients with suprarenal aneurysms or aortic aneurysms requiring repair of associated, clinically significant renal artery occlusive disease (Table 1).

Thus, because of the emerging importance of the appropriate management and anticipated outcome of pararenal aortic aneurysm repair, and the current lack of published data regarding the results of treatment for pararenal aortic aneurysm repair, we recently reviewed the outcome of 257 consecutive patients treated at UCSF.[16] The purpose of the review was to determine the current results of standard open operative management of the 3 patterns of pararenal aortic aneurysm disease. Included in this review were all patients who underwent repair of an aortic aneurysm, requiring

TABLE 1.
Patient Demographics

	JR-AAA (N = 122)		SR-AAA (N = 58)		AAA + RAOD (N = 77)	
	N	%	N	%	N	%
Age (years)*	70.5 ± 8.3		67.6 ± 8.2		67.5 ± 9.3	
Gender						
Men	97	79.5	46	79.3	44	57.1
Woment	25	20.5	12	20.7	33	42.9
Coronary artery disease	73	59.8	31	53.4	35	45.5
Diabetes	8	6.6	4	6.9	13	16.9
Smoking history	101	82.8	50	86.2	59	76.6
Hypertension†	75	61.5	36	62.1	70	90.9

*P less than .05 (analysis of variance [ANOVA]).
†P less than .05 (chi-square).
Abbreviations: JR-AAA, Juxtarenal abdominal aortic aneurysm; *SR-AAA,* suprarenal AAA; *RAOD,* renal artery occlusive disease.
(Courtesy of Jean-Claude JM, Reilly LM, Stoney RJ, et al: Pararenal aortic aneurysms: The future of open aortic repair. *J Vasc Surg* 29:902-912, 1999.)

placement of the aortic crossclamp proximal to the renal arteries. The aortic crossclamp was proximal to all renal arteries in 78.2% of the patients in the study. No patients who underwent aortic reconstruction for aortic occlusive disease or whose aortic aneurysms were repaired with an infrarenal clamp, or who had type IV thoracoabdominal and ruptured AAAs were included. During the first decade of analysis, clinical data were obtained by retrospective review. However, for the last decade, data were collected prospectively, including indications for operations, size of aneurysm, details of operative management, crossclamp level, length of renal ischemia, length of visceral ischemia, and intraoperative and postoperative complications.

PATIENTS

The study group was composed of 122 patients who required suprarenal crossclamping for repair of an infrarenal aneurysm (juxtarenal aneurysm group, JR-AAA) (Fig 1), 58 patients who required renal artery reconstruction to repair an aneurysm extending above the renal arteries (suprarenal aneurysm group, SR-AAA) (Fig 2), and 77 patients with a juxtarenal aortic aneurysm and associated symptomatic renal atherosclerosis (juxtarenal aneurysm and

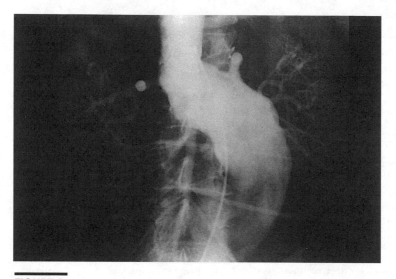

FIGURE 1.

Juxtarenal abdominal aortic aneurysm. No normal aorta exists below the renal arteries to allow deployment of an endovascular device. Repair requires a suprarenal aortic crossclamp, but the proximal anastomosis can be placed immediately below the renal artery orifices. (Courtesy of Jean-Claude JM, Reilly LM, Stoney RJ, et al: Pararenal aortic aneurysms: The future of open aortic repair. *J Vasc Surg* 29:902-912, 1999.)

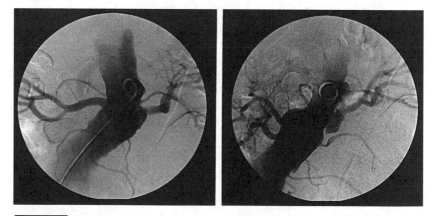

FIGURE 2.

Anterior **(left)** and oblique **(right)** views of suprarenal abdominal aortic aneurysm. Repair requires reconstruction of both renal arteries, due to aneurysmal degeneration of the pararenal aorta. (Courtesy of Jean-Claude JM, Reilly LM, Stoney RJ, et al: Pararenal aortic aneurysms: The future of open aortic repair. *J Vasc Surg* 29:902-912, 1999.)

renal artery occlusive disease group, AAA+RAOD) (Fig 3). Certain demographic features of these patients are worthy of note (Table 1). The mean age was 68.9 ± 8.7 years, and patients in the JR-AAA group were older than patients in the other 2 groups. Most patients were men (n = 187, 73.8%), although the frequency of women was significantly higher in the AAA+RAOD group than in the other 2 groups. The frequency of most risk factors for atherosclerosis was similar among the groups except for hypertension, which occurred significantly more often in the AAA+RAOD group (Table 1). Not surprisingly, patients in this group also had a significantly higher inci-

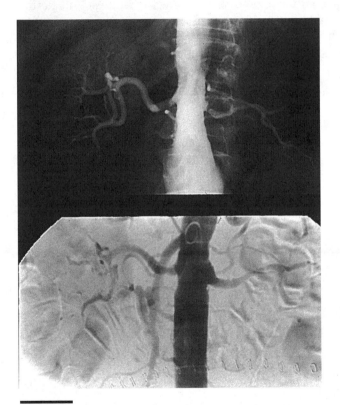

FIGURE 3.
Upper panel, Juxtarenal abdominal aortic aneurysm and severe renal artery occlusive disease. Although not well demonstrated on this angiogram, computed tomography showed the aneurysm to extend to the level of the renal arteries. **Lower panel,** Postoperative angiogram after suprarenal aortic crossclamp, transaortic renal endarterectomy, and infrarenal aortic grafting. (Courtesy of Jean-Claude JM, Reilly LM, Stoney RJ, et al: Pararenal aortic aneurysms: The future of open aortic repair. *J Vasc Surg* 29:902-912, 1999.)

dence of impaired renal function *preoperatively* (serum creatinine, 1.5 mg/dL) (Table 2). The mean diameter of the aortic aneurysms in this study population (6.7 cm ± 2.1 cm) was larger than that typically seen in referral-based studies of infrarenal aneurysms. The patients requiring simultaneous renal artery revascularization had significantly smaller aneurysms than did the other 2 groups (Table 3).

OPERATIVE TECHNIQUE

Successful management of pararenal aortic aneurysm repair requires a thorough knowledge of the anatomy of the proximal aorta and accurate interpretation of preoperative imaging studies. This permits identification of an appropriate site for the proximal aortic anastomosis as well as the method of visceral and renal revascularization. Our 2 most common operative approaches were the standard transperitoneal-infracolic aortic exposure (n = 192, 74.7%) and medial visceral rota-

TABLE 2.
Renal Function Data

	JR-AAA (N = 122)		SR-AAA (N = 58)		AAA + RAOD (N = 77)	
	N	%	N	%	N	%
Renal Function						
Admission*						
Abnormal	27	22.1	14	24.1	39	50.6
Postoperative						
Transient Cr rise	38	31.1	22	37.9	18	23.4
Sustained Cr rise	9	7.3	7	12.1	8	10.4
New-onset dialysis	7	5.7	5	8.6	6	7.8
Dialysis at discharge	1	0.8	3	5.2	3	3.9
Discharge*						
Worse	15	12.3	17	29.3	13	16.9
Improved/unchanged	107	87.7	40	69.0	64	83.1
Serum Cr (mg/dL)						
Preoperative†	1.3 ± 1.0		1.3 ± 0.5		1.9 ± 1.2	
Discharge†	1.6 ± 1.4		1.9 ± 1.6		2.1 ± 1.7	

*P less than .05 (chi-square).
†P less than .05 (ANOVA).
Abbreviations: JR-AAA, Juxtarenal abdominal aortic aneurysm; *SR-AAA,* suprarenal AAA; *RAOD,* renal artery occlusive disease; *Cr,* creatinine.
(Courtesy of Jean-Claude JM, Reilly LM, Stoney RJ, et al: Pararenal aortic aneurysms: The future of open aortic repair. *J Vasc Surg* 29:902-912, 1999.)

TABLE 3.
Operative Data

	JR-AAA (N = 122)		SR-AAA (N = 58)		AAA + RAOD (N = 77)	
	N	%	N	%	N	%
Operation status						
Urgent*	23	18.9	9	15.5	4	5.2
Redo	11	9.0	12	20.7	8	10.4
AAA size (cm)†	7.1 ± 2.1		6.9 ± 2.1		5.9 ± 1.7	
Aortic graft type						
Tube	48	39.3	23	39.7	32	41.6
Aortoiliac	62	50.8	29	50.0	36	46.8
Aortofemoral	7	5.7	5	8.6	9	11.7
Aortoiliofemoral	5	4.1	1	1.7	0	0.0
Renal reconstruction type*						
Bypass	N/A		12	20.7	3	3.9
Reimplantation	N/A		37	63.8	0	0.0
Endarterectomy	N/A		1	1.7	71	92.2
Renal arteries repaired*						
Unilateral	N/A		32	55.2	34	44.2
Bilateral	N/A		15	25.9	40	51.9
Unilateral-accessory	N/A		8	13.8	3	3.9
Bilateral-accessory	N/A		3	5.2	0	0.0
Cross-clamp level*						
Supraceliac	14	11.5	17	29.3	2	2.6
Supra-SMA	7	5.8	28	22.4	28	36.4
Suprarenal	100	82.0	13	48.3	46	59.7
Approach						
Standard infracolic	94	77.1	38	65.5	60	77.9
Medial visceral rotation	17	13.9	13	22.4	12	15.6
EBL (L)	3.8 ± 4.7		4.5 ± 3.2		3.6 ± 5.5	
Length of ischemia (minutes)						
Renal†	27.7 ± 10.6		43.6 ± 38.9		28.7 ± 9.7	
Visceral	35.3 ± 14.6		35.3 ± 14.1		29.0 ± 9.0	

*P less than .05 (chi-square)
†P less than .05 (ANOVA)
Abbreviations: JR-AAA, Juxtarenal abdominal aortic aneurysm; *SR-AAA,* suprarenal AAA; *RAOD,* renal artery occlusive disease; *N/A,* not applicable; *SMA,* superior mesenteric artery; *EBL,* estimated blood loss.
(Courtesy of Jean-Claude JM, Reilly LM, Stoney RJ, et al: Pararenal aortic aneurysms: The future of open aortic repair. *J Vasc Surg* 29:902-912, 1999.)

tion (n = 42, 16.3%). The retroperitoneal, thoracoretroperitoneal, and thoracoabdominal approaches were used rarely.

The transperitoneal-infracolic aortic exposure is performed through a standard full-length abdominal incision extending from just at or above the xyphoid process to the pubic symphysis and was used in 77.1% of the JR-AAA patients and 77.9% of the AAA+RAOD patients. Medial visceral rotation was performed from the left side after full-length midline abdominal incisions. The technique of medial visceral rotation usually included mobilization of all the abdominal viscera (colon, pancreas, stomach, spleen), but can be modified to include only the colon, including the splenic flexure for a partial or limited medial visceral rotation, depending on the extent of aortic exposure required. This mobilization is initiated by incising the lateral attachments of the sigmoid and descending colon, spleen, and gastroesophageal junction. The mobilization of the abdominal viscera can be developed either anterior or posterior to the left kidney. Factors influencing the decision to rotate the left kidney include the extent of aortic aneurysmal dilatation of the paravisceral aorta and the need for concomitant endarterectomy. A medial visceral rotation was used to provide aortic exposure most often in the SR-AAA group (Table 3).

The key additional elements required for adequate exposure of the pararenal aorta include management of the left renal vein, the periaortic ganglionic tissue, and the diaphragmatic crus. Full mobilization of the left renal vein opens the paravisceral aorta for dissection. The left renal vein is mobilized circumferentially from the confluence of the renal vein branches in the hilum of the kidney to its junction with the inferior vena cava, so that it can be widely retracted as needed. This usually requires sacrifice of the adrenal vein, the ascending lumbar branch vein, and the gonadal vein. Such wide mobilization of the left renal vein makes transection of the left renal vein unnecessary. If one wishes to consider the latter option, this decision should be made before sacrifice of the renal vein branches, so that they may provide collateral outflow channels. Occasionally it is necessary to sacrifice 1 or 2 lumbar branches of the vena cava to obtain wide exposure of the right renal artery. After wide mobilization of the left renal vein, the paravisceral aorta is exposed by excising the dense autonomic ganglia from the anterolateral surface of the aorta. The third step is to divide the tendinous portion of the crus of the diaphragm on both sides of the aorta to open completely the periaortic space and allow for safe *vertical* placement of the aortic clamp. Thus, it is not necessary to obtain full circumferential mobilization of the suprarenal or supravisceral aorta, as is usually the case for infrarenal aortic crossclamping. The maintenance of this exposure is facilitated greatly by use of a self-retaining retraction system (eg, Omnitract, Minneapolis, Minn).

OPERATIVE RESULTS

Most of the operative procedures were elective (n = 221, 86.0%). The frequency of urgent procedures was significantly lower in the AAA+RAOD group in comparison with the other 2 groups (Table 3). In 31 cases (12.1%), the patient had a prior aortic reconstruction. Although there were more aortic reoperations in the SR-AAA group, this difference did not achieve significance at the .05 level. Suprarenal aortic crossclamping was applied in 159 patients (61.9%) and was used most often in the JR-AAA group. In 63 patients, supra–superior mesenteric artery (SMA) aortic clamping was used, and was most common in the AAA+RAOD group. Supraceliac aortic clamping was necessary in only 33 patients (12.8%), and was most common in the SR-AAA group (Table 3). Approximately 90% of the patients underwent aortoiliac grafting (n = 127, 49.4%) or an aorto-aortic interposition graft (n = 103, 40.1%). All 3 groups were identical in this regard. The most common technique used for renal artery revascularization in the SR-AAA group was reimplantation (n = 37, 63.8%), whereas the most common method in the AAA+RAOD group was transaortic endarterectomy (n = 71, 92.2%). These differences are significant and reflected the involvement of the renal arteries by the aneurysm in the SR-AAA group and the presence of renal artery occlusive lesions in the AAA+RAOD group. Bilateral renal revascularization was performed in 55 patients (40.7%), and was significantly more common in the AAA+RAOD group. Unilateral renal artery repair was accomplished in 66 patients (48.9%), and was more common in the SR-AAA group. Accessory renal arteries alone required revascularization in 14 patients (10.3%). The average blood loss was 3.9 ± 4.6 L; it did not vary between groups. The duration of renal ischemia (for the supra-SMA or supraceliac aortic crossclamps) averaged 32.9 ± 12.9 minutes, and the average duration of renal ischemia was 31.6 ± 21.6 minutes. Renal ischemia was significantly longer in the SR-AAA group, in comparison with the other 2 groups (Table 3).

OUTCOME

The overall mortality rate was 5.8% (3 intraoperative and 12 postoperative deaths), and no differences were found between groups

(Table 4). The 3 intraoperative deaths and 1 of the postoperative deaths were secondary to the consequences of bleeding. Additionally, 1 patient died of a myocardial infarction, 1 of a saddle pulmonary embolus, 1 of sepsis probably related to endocarditis, and 1 of progressive hepatic failure, related to underlying hepatitis, not to ischemia. One patient died of multisystem organ failure, related to previously undiagnosed metastatic lung cancer. The remaining 6 patients all died of the consequences of postoperative visceral ischemia and infarction, making this the most common cause of death in this study group. Among these 6 patients, 2 had supraceliac crossclamp, 3 supra-SMA, and 1 suprarenal. The involved segment of the gastrointestinal tract was the colon in 2 patients, small bowel in 1, and both in the remaining 3 patients. The underlying cause was embolization in 4 cases, thrombosis in 1, and was uncertain in the final patient.

Regression analysis of perioperative factors indicated that intraoperative bleeding, postoperative visceral ischemia or infarction, and postoperative hematologic complications (bleeding) were significantly correlated with mortality. Type of pararenal aneurysm, crossclamp level, myocardial infarction, new-onset dialysis, and pulmonary complications were *not* correlated with mortality.

In general, the type and frequency of complications in this patient group was typical of that for patients undergoing complex

TABLE 4.
Mortality and Morbidity

	N	%
Death	15	5.8
Complications		
Respiratory insufficiency	19	7.4
Pneumonia	15	5.8
Myocardial infarction	15	5.8
Stroke	5	1.9
Paraplegia	1	0.4
Visceral ischemia/infarction	7	2.7
Lower limb embolization	9	3.5
Lower limb thrombosis requiring reoperation	7	2.7
Wound infection	5	1.9
Wound dehiscence	4	1.6

(Courtesy of Jean-Claude JM, Reilly LM, Stoney RJ, et al: Pararenal aortic aneurysms: The future of open aortic repair. *J Vasc Surg* 29:902-912, 1999.)

aortic reconstruction. The most common postoperative complications were pulmonary complications (n = 37, 14.4%; Table 4). Of these pulmonary complications, pneumonia (n = 15) and respiratory failure requiring prolonged intubation (n = 19) were the most common. Infectious complications were second in frequency (n = 36, 14.0%). The most frequent site of infection was in the lungs (pneumonia, n = 15), followed by intra-abdominal infections related to visceral ischemia or infarction (n = 7), urinary tract infections (n = 6), and wound infections (n = 5). Myocardial complications occurred in 13.2% of patients (n = 34), usually arrhythmias (n = 16) or myocardial infarction (n = 15). Only one perioperative MI was fatal, a surprising finding. One of the 14 nonfatal myocardial infarctions occurred in a patient who died, but it was not the cause of his death. Nineteen patients (7.4%) had vascular complications: lower extremity thrombosis, embolization, or compartment syndrome (n = 10), visceral artery thrombosis (n = 1), renal artery bypass thrombosis (n = 1), and deep venous thrombosis (n = 3). Twenty-one patients underwent reoperations (8.2%), most commonly for lower extremity arterial thrombosis/embolization/compartment syndrome (n = 7), or for visceral ischemia or infarction (n = 6). Wound complications occurred in 10 patients (3.8%), including infection (n = 5) and dehiscence (n = 4), and 3 of these required reoperation for reclosure. Neurologic complications occurred in 16 patients (16.2%), including 5 strokes and transient ischemia attacks. Only 1 patient developed paraplegia (0.3%), and no differences were noted between groups in frequency of these complications.

The major concern for patients undergoing pararenal aortic aneurysm repair is the effect of the period of obligatory renal ischemia on renal function. Some elevation of serum creatinine levels (> 0.5 mg/dL) occurred in 102 patients (40.5%; Table 2). Eighteen patients (17%) required dialysis in the postoperative period; 7 had suprarenal crossclamps, 5 had a supra-SMA, and 6 had supraceliac aortic crossclamps. The average duration of renal ischemia for patients who required postoperative dialysis was 42.1 ± 32.8 minutes, significantly longer than that for patients who did not require dialysis (30.7 ± 20.3 minutes). In terms of the effect of preoperative renal insufficiency on the frequency of postoperative dialysis, patients who required dialysis had an average preoperative creatinine level of 1.8 ± 1.2 mg/dL, not significantly different from the average creatinine level for patients who did not require dialysis (1.5 ± 1.0 mg/dL). Seven of the 18 patients who required postoperative dialysis no longer did so at the time of discharge; 3

normalized their creatinine levels to the preoperative levels, whereas 4 others had some persistent elevation of their serum creatinine. The remaining 11 patients continue to require dialysis at the time of discharge (n = 7), or at their death (n = 4), yielding an incidence of new permanent dialysis of 4.3%.

Eighty-six patients (33.5%) had an increase in serum creatinine level of greater than 0.5 mg/dL, but did not require dialysis. At discharge, 55 of these patients returned to their baseline level while 29 had not (no data in 2 patients). At discharge, the creatinine level had decreased from its postoperative maximum in 16 of these 29 patients, but stayed within 0.5 mg/dL of the postoperative maximum in the remaining 13 patients. Thus, of 104 patients with some increase in serum creatinine levels in the postoperative period, by the time of discharge or death, 58 (56%) of these patients had returned to their preoperative serum creatinine levels, including 3 who had required dialysis. An additional 20 patients (19%) had improving renal function but had not yet reached their preoperative baseline levels, including 4 who had required dialysis; 13 patients (12.5%) remained worse with no clear improvement, and 11 patients (10.6%) remained on dialysis. No difference between the 3 treatment groups in the frequency of postoperative renal insufficiency or new-onset dialysis was observed. Persistent elevation of the serum creatinine level at the time discharge occurred more often in the SR-AAA group, a significant difference in comparison with the JR-AAA group, but not in comparison with the AAA+RAOD group (Table 2). When regression analysis was used to identify factors correlating with renal morbidity, only preoperative renal functional status and duration of renal ischemia were significant. Neither aortic crossclamp level nor type of renal reconstruction correlated with loss of renal function or requirement for dialysis.

ANALYSIS

One general assumption concerning the cause and risk of death after repair of pararenal aneurysms is that cardiac complications such as myocardial infarction and serious arrhythmias would play a substantial role in outcome. Somewhat surprisingly, this was not the case in the UCSF experience. Death from myocardial infarction accounted for only 1 (6.7%) of 15 deaths. In contrast, in other published series that contained patients with comparable patterns of pararenal aneurysms, myocardial infarction accounted for 40% of deaths (8 of 20). A number of factors may have contributed to the low cardiac morbidity in this study. First, we obtain selective preoperative cardiac evaluation in patients with clinically significant coronary artery disease. Intraoperatively, transesophageal echocardiography is used regularly. Transesophageal echocardiography provides real-time assessment of cardiac function and, perhaps more importantly, identifies onset of new segmental wall motion abnormalities coincident with intraoperative ischemia that can be treated and reversed before causing clinical complications. In addition, it is a highly reliable way in which to determine the adequacy of intravascular volume. Although intraoperative pulmonary artery wedge pressures can be obtained, the frequent intraoperative changes in myocardial compliance distort the significance between the pulmonary artery wedge pressure and left atrial pressure. Thus, we rely heavily on transesophageal echocardiography for intraoperative assessment and management of cardiac function and volume status. A third potentially critical factor that may have led to a reduced rate of fatal myocardial infarctions is the limited use of supraceliac aortic crossclamping (13% of cases). In many of the other series of pararenal aneurysm repair, supraceliac clamping was used predominantly or exclusively.[7,9,11,13,14] Supraceliac aortic crossclamping places a substantial stress on the myocardium and has been shown to induce acute segmental wall changes and myocardial dysfunction in up to 20% of patients.[9,17] In addition, avoidance of supraceliac aortic clamping reduces the frequency of hepatic ischemia and the attendant effects of an increase in fibrinolysis and thereby potential bleeding complications. Finally, routine supraceliac aortic crossclamping may unnecessarily increase the duration of renal ischemia. Thus, the combined use of transesophageal echocardiography and minimal supraceliac aortic occlusion minimizes intraoperative myocardial injury and may be largely responsible for the reduced rate and severity of cardiac morbidity noted in our experience.

Visceral ischemia or infarction was the primary cause of death in our patients (6 of 15, 40%) and was an unexpected finding. Intraoperative mesenteric embolization occurred in at least 4 and possibly 5 of these patients. In the remaining patient, underestimation of the severity of occlusive lesions in the celiac artery and the SMA resulted in postoperative thrombosis. Among deaths reported in other series of pararenal aortic aneurysm repairs, only 3 deaths (7.5%) were attributed to visceral ischemia or infarction. One possibility is that mobilization and crossclamping of the pararenal or para-SMA aorta may increase the risk of embolization.[9,13] Others have recommended avoiding the para-SMA aorta entirely and routinely using the supraceliac aorta for clamp placement because of the less frequent involvement of this area with atherosclerosis and greater ease of mobilization of the supraceliac aorta.[8,9,13,14] An important point in this regard is that the 2 series with the greatest use of supra-SMA crossclampling (18%)[11,16] demonstrated no correlation between aortic crossclamp level and patient outcome. Perhaps of greater importance in the UCSF series, no correlation between crossclamp level and the development of visceral ischemia or infarction was found. Thus, with increasing experience, exposure of the pararenal and paravisceral aorta, and knowledge of its key elements play an important role in reducing such complications. Looking to the future, efforts to reduce further the incidence of atheroembolization should include careful preoperative assessment of the extent of aortic disease at the planned level of crossclamping, selection of the optimal approach for the required exposure, and following the proper clamping and declamping sequence for the aorta and visceral branches.

The frequency of renal dysfunction, defined as an increase of the serum creatinine level by more than 0.5 mg/dL over preoperative values, was 40.5%. This is a higher rate of renal dysfunction than that observed in other series of pararenal aneurysm repair (Table 5). However, of equal importance is the 31% incidence of abnormal baseline renal function in the patients in the UCSF experience. It is also the highest reported rate, and preoperative renal function status was correlated significantly with the incidence of postoperative renal insufficiency. Allen et al[11] also reported that preoperative renal insufficiency was a significant factor for postoperative decline in renal function, although other investigators[12,13] reported no such correlation. The rate of temporary or permanent dialysis in this series (7%), as well as the rate of some renal functional impairment at discharge or death (10.5%), is within the range reported by others (Table 5). The pattern of renal insufficiency noted in this series was most consistent with a mechanism of acute tubular necrosis that occurred as a result of the duration of crossclamp-induced renal ischemia and other perioperative physiologic changes impairing renal perfusion. It is not likely to be related to atheroembolization. The rapid onset as well as the rapid resolution in most patients who have renal insufficiency is most consistent with acute tubular necrosis as an etiology. Long-term reassessment of these patients' renal function during late follow-up will be important in further defining the mechanism of postoperative changes in renal function in patients undergoing pararenal aortic aneurysm repair.

As might be expected, the duration of renal ischemia correlated

TABLE 5.
Literature Summary

Study	N	AAA Type*	Cross-clamp Level	Mortality	Baseline Elevated Cr	Transient Cr Rise	New-onset Dialysis	Elevated Cr at Discharge
Crawford et al 1986	101	JR = 88 SR = 0 RAOD = 13	SC = 93 SSMA = 0 SR = 8	7.9%	18.8%	15.8%	7.9%	ND
Qvarfordt et al 1986	77	JR = 22 SR = 24 RAOD = 31	SC = 13 SSMA = 17 SR = 45	1.3%	54.5%	23.0%	2.5%	13.0%
Green et al† 1989	52	JR = 29 SR = ? RAOD = ?	SC = 30 SSMA = 0 SR = 22	15.4%	ND	ND	11.5%	ND
Poulias et al 1992	38	JR = 32 SR = 0 RAOD = 6	SC = 0 SSMA = 0 SR = 38	5.3%	15.8%	23.7%	13.2%	13.2%
Breckwoldt et al‡ 1992	39	Unclear	SC = 8 SSMA = 2 SR = 25	2.6%	ND	28.2%	2.6%	12.8%
Allen et al§ 1993	65	JR = 24 SR = 15 RAOD = 7	SC = 27 SSMA = 12 SR = 26	1.5%	20.0%	12.3%	3.1%	3.1%

(continued)

TABLE 5. (continued)

Study	N	AAA Type*	Cross-clamp Level	Mortality	Baseline Elevated Cr	Transient Cr Rise	New-onset Dialysis	Elevated Cr at Discharge
Nypaver et al 1993	53	JR = 41 SR = 6 RAOD = 6	SC = 21 SSMA = 4 SR = 28	3.8%	17.0%	22.6%	5.7%	7.5%
Schneider et al 1997	23	JR = 23 SR = 0 RAOD = 0	SC = 23 SSMA = 0 SR = 0	0.0%	ND	26.1%	0.0%	0.0%
Faggioli et al[||] 1998	50	JR = 39 SR = 6 RAOD = 5	SC = 8 SSMA = 0 SR = 42	7.0% (elective only)	10.0%	ND	ND	0.0%
Jean-Claude et al 1999	257	JR = 122 SR = 58 RAOD = 77	SC = 33 SSMA = 48 SR = 174	5.8%	31.1%	30.4%	7.0%	10.5%

*Best estimate of categorization using UCSF pararenal AAA groups.

†Very difficult to put the data in this study into this format; also SR clamp group contains 11 patients who initially had an infrarenal clamp.

‡Only 33 AAAs match UCSF categories.

§Only 46 AAAs match UCSF categories.

||Includes 7 ruptured pararenal AAAs.

Abbreviations: AAA, Abdominal aortic aneurysm; *Cr*, creatinine; *JR*, juxtarenal AAA; *SR*, suprarenal AAA; *RAOD*, renal artery occlusive disease + AAA; *SC*, supraceliac; *SSMA*, supra-superior mesenteric artery; *ND*, no clear data.

(Courtesy of Jean-Claude JM, Reilly LM, Stoney RJ, et al: Pararenal aortic aneurysms: The future of open aortic repair. *J Vasc Surg* 29:902-912, 1999.)

with an increased risk of loss of renal function postoperatively. A number of techniques can be used to minimize the duration of renal ischemia. First, the aortic clamp is always positioned in such a manner as to preserve flow to some renal parenchyma when that is possible. This was anatomically possible in only 22% of the patients in this group. Second, the aortic clamp is repositioned onto the prosthetic graft as soon as the proximal anastomosis is completed. Third, for SR-AAA patients, whenever possible, a beveled proximal aortic anastomosis is performed, incorporating one of the renal orifices. This technique restores perfusion to one of the kidneys rapidly and leaves only one artery to be reimplanted or grafted. Fourth, for the AAA+RAOD patients, transaortic endarterectomy is the most expeditious method to treat the occlusive disease affecting both kidneys, and particularly when there are multiple renal arteries.

Other groups have recommended hypothermic renal profusion as a protective mechanism, which extends the ischemic tolerance of the renal parenchyma by reducing its metabolic rate.[11] Cold renal prefusion was used selectively in the UCSF series (27% of the patients). For the JR-AAA group, the aortic crossclamp time is so short that cold perfusion will rarely be of benefit. In the AAA+RAOD group, endarterectomy was used to treat the renal occlusive lesions simultaneously, thus obviating the use of cold perfusion in this group as well. Cold renal perfusion was used most commonly in the SR-AAA group in whom the duration of renal ischemia is the longest, particularly for the left kidney if it is not incorporated in the proximal anastomosis. The use of cold renal perfusion in published series of pararenal aneurysm repair varies widely.[11-14] Usually, its use is based on the anticipated duration of renal ischemia and the preoperative renal functional status. Our current standard for minimizing renal ischemia is to monitor urine output at 15-minute intervals throughout the operative period; to use felodipine, which is a selective renal vasodilator and for which there is increasing evidence that it is highly effective in reducing complications of renal ischemia; and to administer 12.5 g of mannitol before and after the induction of renal ischemia. We continue the felodipine for 24 hours or longer depending on the duration of renal ischemia. Furthermore, we avoid the use of any iodinated contrast studies in the 48 hours before the planned operative procedure.

CONCLUSIONS

Pararenal aortic aneurysms can be treated safely and effectively, with morbidity and mortality rates that approach those of standard infrarenal aortic aneurysm repair. This is dependent on appropriate preoperative patient assessment including selective optimization of cardiac function, optimal selection of operative strategy, careful intraoperative anesthetic management including the use of transesophageal echocardiography, meticulous attention to operative technical detail, and skilled postoperative management. The outcome for the 3 patterns of pararenal aortic aneurysmal disease is similar, but preoperative abnormal renal function, particularly in combination with a prolonged interval of renal ischemia, is associated with an increased risk of further loss of renal function. We believe these results provide a reference point for the expected treatment outcomes in patients with these patterns of pararenal aortic aneurysmal disease, which currently can be managed only by open surgical repair.

REFERENCES

1. Chuter TAM, Green RM, Ouriel K, et al: Infrarenal aortic aneurysm structure: Implications for transfemoral repair. *J Vasc Surg* 20:44-50, 1994.
2. Ernst CB: Abdominal aortic aneurysm. *N Engl J Med* 328:1167-1172, 1993.
3. Katz DJ, Stanley JC, Zelenock GB: Operative mortality rates for intact and ruptured abdominal aortic aneurysms in Michigan: An eleven-year statewide experience. *J Vasc Surg* 19:804-817, 1994.
4. Pearce WH, Feinglass J, Sohn M-W, et al: Hospital vascular surgery volume and procedure mortality rates in California, 1982-1994. *J Vasc Surg* 29:768-776, 1999.
5. Kazmers A, Jacobs L, Perkins A, et al: Abdominal aortic aneurysm repair in Veterans Affairs medical centers. *J Vasc Surg* 23:191-200, 1996.
6. Johnston KW, Scobie TK: Multicenter prospective study of nonruptured abdominal aortic aneurysms: I. Population and operative management. *J Vasc Surg* 7:69-81, 1988.
7. Crawford ES, Beckett WC, Greer MS: Juxtarenal infrarenal abdominal aortic aneurysm. Special diagnostic and therapeutic considerations. *Ann Surg* 203:661-670, 1986.
8. Qvarfordt PG, Stoney RJ, Reilly LM, et al: Management of pararenal aneurysm of the abdominal aorta. *J Vasc Surg* 3:84- 93, 1986.
9. Green RM, Ricotta JJ, Ouriel K, et al: Results of supraceliac aortic clamping in the difficult elective resection of infrarenal abdominal aortic aneurysm. *J Vasc Surg* 9:125-134, 1989.
10. Poulias GE, Doundoulatis N, Skoutas B, et al: Juxtarenal aortic aneurysmectomy. *J Cardiovasc Surg* 33:324-330, 1992.
11. Allen BT, Anderson CB, Rubin BG, et al: Preservation of renal function in juxtarenal and suprarenal abdominal aortic aneurysm repair. *J Vasc Surg* 17:948-959, 1993.
12. Breckwoldt WL, Mackey WC, Belkin M, et al: The effect of suprarenal

crossclamping on abdominal aortic aneurysm repair. *Arch Surg* 127:520-524, 1992.

13. Nypaver TJ, Shepard AD, Reddy DJ, et al: Repair of pararenal abdominal aortic aneurysms. An analysis of operative management. *Arch Surg* 128:803-813, 1993.

14. Schneider JR, Gottner RJ, Golan JF: Supraceliac versus infrarenal aortic cross-clamp for repair of non-ruptured infrarenal and juxtarenal abdominal aortic aneurysm. *Cardiovasc Surg* 5:279-285, 1997.

15. Faggioli G, Stella A, Freyrie A, et al: Early and long- term results in the surgical treatment of juxtarenal and pararenal aortic aneurysms. *Eur J Vasc Endovasc Surg* 15:205-211, 1998.

16. Jean-Claude JM, Reilly LM, Stoney RJ, et al: Pararenal aortic aneurysms: The future of open aortic aneurysm repair. *J Vasc Surg* 29:902-912, 1999.

17. Rosen MF, Beauport PN, Alert RA, et al: Monitoring with two-dimensional transesophageal echocardiography. *J Vasc Surg* 1:300-305, 1984.

CHAPTER 4

Endovascular Grafts for Ruptured Aneurysms*

Takao Ohki, MD
Assistant Professor of Surgery, Albert Einstein College of Medicine,
Chief, Endovascular Program, Montefiore Medical Center, New York

Frank J. Veith, MD
Professor of Surgery, Albert Einstein College of Medicine, Chief,
Vascular Surgical Services, Montefiore Medical Center, New York

Maseet A. Bade, MD
Research Fellow in Vascular Surgery, Montefiore Medical Center, New York

Lu Zhan, BS
Medical Student, Albert Einstein College of Medicine, New York

Four decades have passed since the first successful repair of an infrarenal abdominal aortic aneurysm (AAA) was reported. During this period, several important advances have been made in the nonsurgical aspect of care. These include the transportation of patients with ruptured AAAs, their critical care, management of their cardiac dysfunction, and pharmacologic support. In spite of these efforts, operative mortality rates have not improved significantly and still range from 24% to 70%.[1-16] In part, this is because the basic surgical techniques for repairing ruptured AAAs remain little changed, although a number of minor improvements have been introduced. These minor improvements include supraceliac clamping, suturing the graft within the aneurysm without excising it, more frequent use of tube grafts, and use of lower porosity prostheses.[2,3,5,6,8-10,12] However, general anesthesia, the large surgical incision, the amount of dissection, and the accompanying invasiveness and blood loss required for open repair have largely remained unchanged and may be responsible for the poor outcome.

*Supported by grants from the US Public Health Service (HL 02990-04), the James Hilton Manning and Emma Austin Manning Foundation, and the Anne S. Brown Trust.

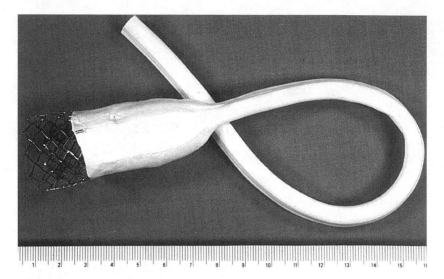

FIGURE 1.

The Vascular Innovation graft. An extra large Palmaz stent is attached to the polytetrafluoroethylene (PTFE) graft.

INHERENT LIMITATIONS AND POTENTIAL BENEFITS OF ENDOVASCULAR GRAFT REPAIR FOR RUPTURED ANEURYSMS

Endovascular grafts (EVGs) have been used to treat a variety of arterial pathologies, including elective AAAs, iliac artery aneurysms, occlusive disease, and traumatic lesions, with promising short- and mid-term results.[17-26] Although EVGs are theoretically appealing because of their minimally invasive nature, their use in the treatment of ruptured AAAs or iliac artery aneurysms had been limited to a single case report.[27] One major reason for this limited use of EVGs in this acute setting has been the need for preoperative measurements of the aneurysmal and adjacent arterial anatomy so that an appropriate size and configuration of graft can be selected, and the resulting delay has been deemed inappropriate in the urgent setting of ruptured AAAs.

EXPERIENCE AT MONTEFIORE MEDICAL CENTER WITH ENDOVASCULAR REPAIR OF RUPTURED AAAS

VASCULAR INNOVATION "ONE SIZE FITS MOST" GRAFT

We developed the Vascular Innovation (VI) graft (Vascular Innovation Inc, Toledo, Ohio), which facilitates intraoperative customization, thus eliminating the need for preoperative measure-

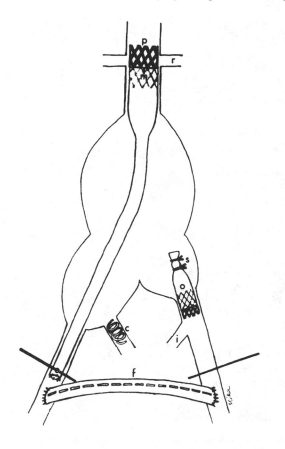

FIGURE 2.

Schematic drawing of how the Vascular Innovation (VI) graft is deployed. The VI graft is fixed within the proximal neck with a large Palmaz stent *(p)*. The cranial end of the graft is denoted by the metallic marker *(m)* attached to the graft. In this example, the bare portion of the stent is deployed across the orifice of the renal arteries so that the graft is implanted immediately below the renal arteries *(r)*. An endoluminal anastomosis *(e)* is performed at the distal end of the EVG. The occluder device *(o)* is always deployed in the contralateral common iliac artery to preserve at least one internal iliac artery *(i)*. *Abbreviations: c,* Embolization coil; *f,* femoro-femoral bypass; *s,* suture to occlude the end of the occluder.

ments and fabrication of the graft.[28,29] The VI graft (Figs 1 and 2) is constructed by suturing a Palmaz stent (P5O14, Cordis, Warren, NJ) to a standard wall expanded polytetrafluoroethylene (ePTFE) graft (6 mm × 40 cm; IMPRA, Tempe, Ariz).[28] This stent-graft combination is mounted onto a large percutaneous transluminal angioplasty (PTA) balloon (Maxi LD, 25 mm × 4 cm; Cordis, Warren, NJ)

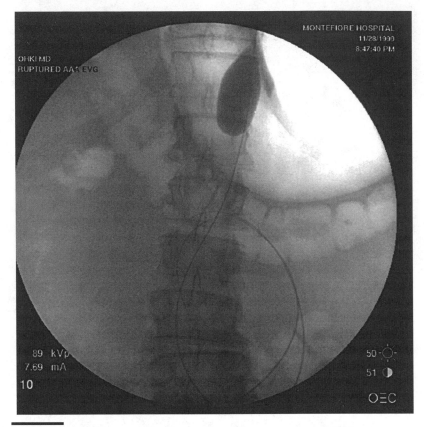

FIGURE 3.
Fluoroscopic view of a brachially introduced proximal occlusion balloon

and then inserted into a 16F Sheath (Cook Inc, Bloomington, Ind). An occluder device (for occlusion of the opposite common iliac artery) is constructed by attaching a Palmaz stent (P4014 or P308) to an ePTFE graft closed at one end by ligatures. This occluder is also mounted onto a PTA balloon and then is inserted into either a 12F or 16F sheath. These grafts are prefabricated and kept sterile for emergent use.

OBTAINING PROXIMAL CONTROL

In patients who are hemodynamically unstable, an occlusion balloon (Occlusion catheter, Meditech, Oakland, NJ) is inserted and inflated in the suprarenal aorta through the brachial artery (Fig 3). This is performed under local anesthesia to maintain vasoconstriction, which is often released with induction of general anes-

TABLE 1.
Exclusion Criteria for Endovascular Repair

1. Pararenal AAAs (neck length shorter than 5 mm)
2. Proximal neck diameter larger than 28 mm
3. Bilateral long iliac artery occlusions
4. Mycotic aneurysm

Abbreviation: AAA, Abdominal aortic aneurysm.

thesia. In many cases, this vasoconstriction is a key function in maintaining the blood pressure above lethal levels.

INDICATIONS FOR ENDOVASCULAR REPAIR

Under general anesthesia, bilateral common femoral arteries are exposed and introducer sheaths are inserted. In those cases in which a preoperative computed tomography (CT) scan or angiogram was not performed, an aortogram is first obtained using the OEC portable fluoroscope (OEC Model 9800, OEC Medical, Salt Lake City, Utah, or BV 300, Philips, The Netherlands) and the Acist contrast power injector system (Acist Medical Systems, Eden Prairie, Minn). A decision is made regarding the feasibility of an endovascular repair. This decision is based on several criteria shown in Table 1.

DEPLOYMENT TECHNIQUE OF VI GRAFT

Coil embolization of the hypogastric artery ipsilateral to the side of VI graft insertion is performed before or after its deployment.[29] The VI graft delivery system is inserted into the aorta over a super stiff wire placed in the ascending thoracic aorta. Once the graft is inserted into the proximal aneurysm neck, the delivery sheath is retracted and an angiogram is repeated with a pig tail catheter introduced via the contralateral femoral artery to confirm appropriate positioning with regard to the renal arteries. Inflation of the deployment balloon expands the stent and fixes the VI graft within the proximal neck. By varying the inflation pressure, the VI graft is able to accommodate a wide range of proximal neck diameters ranging from 15 to 28 mm (Fig 4). The length of the graft is 40 cm in each case so that the distal end of the graft always emerges from the introduction arteriotomy site. The graft is then cut to appropriate length and hand sewn endoluminally within the common femoral or distal external iliac artery (Fig 5). For AAAs, the VI graft is placed within the proximal neck and the occluder device is

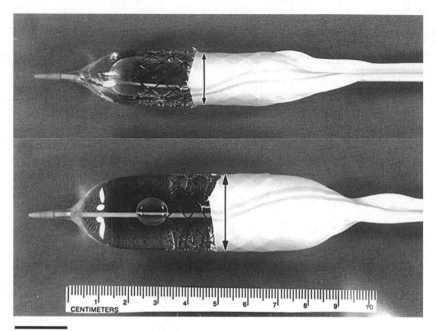

FIGURE 4.
Method of intraoperatively customizing proximal stent diameter of the
Vascular Innovation graft. **A,** When the deployment balloon is inflated to
2 atm, the stent is expanded to 20 mm in diameter *(small arrow)*. **B,** Due
to the compliant nature of the balloon, at 6 atm of inflation pressure, the
stent is expanded to 28 mm *(large arrow)*. (Courtesy of Ohki T, Veith FJ,
Sanchez LA, et al: Endovascular graft repair of ruptured aorto-iliac
aneurysms. *J Am Coll Surg* 189:102-113, 1999. Reprinted with permission
from the American College of Surgeons.)

placed in the opposite common iliac artery, thereby preserving at
least one hypogastric artery. In addition a femoro-femoral bypass
is performed (Figs 6 and 7). For iliac aneurysms with a proximal
common iliac neck, the main EVG is placed from that neck to the
common femoral or external iliac artery.

PATIENTS
Ten patients with ruptured AAAs were treated using the VI graft (9
men). Their mean age was 68 years. The type and location of the
aneurysm included 6 AAAs (5 true, 1 false) and 4 iliac artery
aneurysms (2 true, 2 false). Spiral CT was performed in each case.
All 10 patients were deemed prohibitively high risk for open surgical treatment because of comorbid disease (chronic obstructive
pulmonary disease requiring home oxygen, ejection fraction < 20%

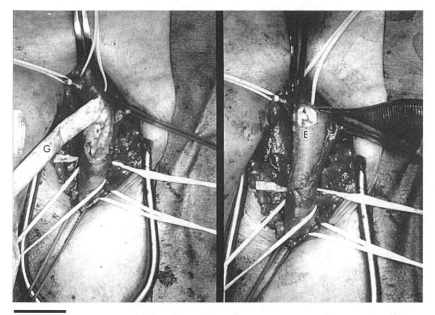

FIGURE 5.

Method of intraoperatively customizing the length of the Vascular Innovation graft. **A,** Each endovascular graft is made long enough so that the distal end of the graft *(G)* emerges from the arteriotomy site in each case. **B,** The graft is cut to the appropriate length as it emerges from the femoral artery. An endoluminal anastomosis *(E)* is carried out. (Courtesy of Ohki T, Veith FJ, Sanchez LA, et al: Endovascular graft repair of ruptured aorto-iliac aneurysms. *J Am Coll Surg* 189:102-113, 1999. Reprinted with permission from the American College of Surgeons.)

[n = 8]) or hostile abdomen (multiple abdominal operations with pelvic irradiation [n = 2]). Seven patients were transferred to our institution from an outside hospital after developing symptoms. In each case, another surgeon considered the patient unsuitable for standard surgery and best treated by an EVG. Preoperative symptoms including acute onset of abdominal or back pain, syncope, or external bleeding were present in all cases. No patient in this series had a cardiac arrest or cardiopulmonary resuscitation preoperatively, although 2 required endotracheal intubation and ventilator support.

OUTCOME

Four cases required rapid proximal arterial control because of sustained hemodynamic instability; control was obtained by the use of a proximal occlusion balloon or by the rapid deployment of the

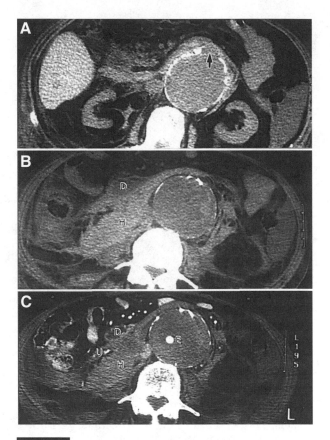

FIGURE 6.
Computed tomography (CT) scan images of a ruptured abdominal aortic aneurysm (AAA). This 71-year-old male was admitted to another hospital for medical treatment of his pneumonia secondary to chemotherapy for leukemia. Other comorbid disease included severe chronic obstructive pulmonary disease (COPD) requiring home oxygen, and congestive heart failure with an ejection fraction of 25%. The patient experienced sudden onset of severe abdominal pain, which was confirmed by CT scan to be a ruptured AAA. Due to his coexisting disease, standard repair was deemed prohibited and he was transferred to our institution. On arrival, his systolic blood pressure was 75 mm Hg and hematocrit was 18%. **A,** Preoperative CT scan reveals possible rupture site *(arrow)* in the AAA. **B,** Preoperative CT scan showing more distal portion of the AAA. The AAA measures 7.5 cm. In addition, a large hematoma *(H)* can be seen in the right retroperitoneal space that is displacing the duodenum *(D).* **C,** Postoperative enhanced CT scan. Contrast is confined within the endovascular graft *(E)* with evidence of complete aneurysmal exclusion. The ureter *(U),* which is displaced by the large hematoma, is visualized. Despite his comorbid condition, he was extubated 6 hours after the procedure and was on a diet on the second postoperative day. (Courtesy of Ohki T, Veith FJ, Sanchez LA, et al: Endovascular graft repair of ruptured aorto-iliac aneurysms. *J Am Coll Surg* 189:102-113, 1999. Reprinted with permission from the American College of Surgeons.)

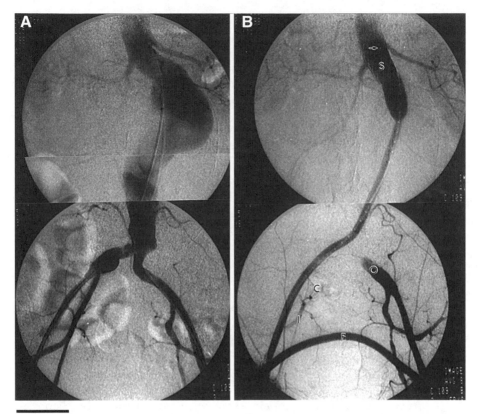

FIGURE 7.

Intraoperative angiogram of the patient described in Figure 5. **A,** Preoperative angiogram reveals large abdominal aortic aneurysm (AAA) and a small common iliac aneurysm. **B,** Completion angiogram. The AAA is completely excluded without an endoleak. The bare portion of the proximal stent *(S)* was placed above the renal arteries and the cranial end of the graft, which is denoted by the gold marker *(arrow)*, is placed immediately below the renal arteries. Right internal iliac artery is opacified by retrograde flow. *Abbreviations: C,* Embolization coils; *I,* internal iliac artery; *O,* occluder device; *F,* femorofemoral bypass. (Courtesy of Ohki T, Veith FJ, Sanchez LA, et al: Endovascular graft repair of ruptured aorto-iliac aneurysms. *J Am Coll Surg* 189:102-113, 1999. Reprinted with permission from the American College of Surgeons.)

EVG. The EVG was successfully deployed at the target site in all cases, with complete exclusion of the ruptured aneurysm and absence of an endoleak. This was accompanied by the resolution of preoperative symptoms in each case. The mean operative time was 5 hours, and the mean blood loss was 800 mL. One patient died in the operating room from cardiac arrest as a result of his pre-existing acute myocardial infarction. Another patient died of multiple organ failure 3 weeks postoperatively. In one case, an evacuation of hematoma was performed through a limited retroperitoneal incision, 7 days postoperatively. There were 3 surgical complications including 1 postoperative myocardial infarction and 2 groin wound infections that required drainage but healed without graft involvement. The mean length of hospital stay was 7 days. One graft occluded 2 months postoperatively, and an axillo-femoral bypass was required. However, this patient's aneurysm continued to be successfully excluded from the circulation until she died from her pre-existing cervical cancer. During the mean follow-up of 15 months, 2 patients died of pre-existing comorbid disease that was unrelated to the EVG repair. In the remaining 6 survivors, there were no signs of endoleak, and each graft continues to be functional at a mean follow-up of 22 months.

COMMENTS

We have developed the VI for which the precise preoperative measurements are largely eliminated. This has been made possible by the use of a compliant stent deployment balloon and by the fact that the graft length is always made longer than required and cut to the proper length in situ as previously described.

One potential disadvantage of EVG repair for ruptured AAAs is that it may take longer to achieve proximal arterial control compared with standard repair. However, if such immediate control was required, we have used an occlusion balloon, which can be inserted from the brachial artery. More liberal use of this technique may further expand the indications for EVG repair in the treatment of ruptured aneurysms.

POTENTIAL ADVANTAGES OF EVG REPAIR IN TREATMENT OF RUPTURED AAAS

There are several potential advantages to EVG repair of ruptured aneurysms. These are summarized below.

1. *Ability to obtain proximal control before general anesthesia induction.* Patients with ruptured AAA may initially be severely hypotensive; however, in many patients, especially those who are able to arrive to the hospital, their blood pressure may be stabilized at a nonlethal level. Stabilization mainly results from vasoconstriction, which is the human body's response to hypotension. It is not rare for the vasoconstriction to be released, on induction of general anesthesia, resulting in a sud-

den decrease in blood pressure. Thus, a relatively stable patient may become severely hypotensive, mandating urgent application of a proximal cross clamping. The use of a cross clamp, as well as the presence of a hematoma that may distort the intra-abdominal anatomy, further poses technical difficulty in the repair of a ruptured AAA. On the other hand, a guide wire can be inserted in the abdominal aorta through a percutaneous puncture under local anesthesia, thereby maintaining the vasoconstriction. Once the guide wire is inserted in the aorta, the patient can safely undergo induction because the proximal control can be rapidly and safely obtained by introducing the brachial occlusion balloon over the previously placed guide wire.

2. *Ability to deploy the graft from a remote access site.* EVGs can be inserted and deployed through a remote access site, thereby obviating the need for laparotomy and more importantly, eliminating the technical difficulties that are encountered when performing a standard repair in this setting. The anatomy of the retroperitoneal structures is often distorted and obscured because of the large hematoma. This may lead not only to technical difficulties but also to inadvertent injury of the inferior vena cava, the left renal vein or its genital branches, the duodenum, and other surrounding structure. These iatrogenic injuries have been the cause of significant operative mortality and morbidity after standard surgery for ruptured aneurysms.[4,6-9,11] In contrast, EVG repair is performed within the arterial tree, which is unaffected by the extravasated blood or from previous operative scarring. Thus, the degree of technical difficulty in treating a ruptured aneurysm with an EVG is almost the same as in elective cases. Moreover, this approach completely eliminates the risk of inadvertent injuries to surrounding structures.

3. *Reduced blood loss.* In our experience, the EVG repair was accomplished with a relatively small amount of blood loss (800 mL) compared with that reported for open ruptured AAA repair. The amount of blood loss during elective EVG repair has also been reported to be less than that accompanying open repair.[30] However, the value of this advantage is far greater in patents with ruptured aneurysms, because these patients have already lost a significant amount of blood after rupture and disseminated intravascular coagulation secondary to blood loss is a devastating complication. Limited blood loss was possible for several reasons, including the fact that EVG repair does not release the tamponade effect within the retroperitoneum and other surrounding structures. In addition, back bleeding from

the iliac and lumbar arteries, bleeding from the anastomotic suture lines, and bleeding from iatrogenic venous injury, which are the main sources of blood loss during standard repair, can be completely eliminated during EVG repair.

4. *Minimizing hypothermia by eliminating laparotomy.* Hypothermia that can be secondary to poor perfusion and laparotomy can exacerbate coagulopathy, which is one of the causes of mortality after surgical repair. EVG can minimize the extent of hypothermia by avoiding laparotomy.

CONCLUSIONS AND FUTURE PROSPECT

Although this study included only high-risk patients all of whom were nonsurgical candidates, the relatively low mortality (20%) and short length of stay (7 days) are encouraging. These results show that EVG repair of ruptured AAAs and iliac artery aneurysms is feasible and effective in selected cases. Further device refinements and longer follow-up are required before widespread use of this technique is adopted. In addition, whether the more liberal use of proximal occlusion balloons will enable the treatment of larger cohorts of patients, including those that are more hemodynamically unstable, remains to be shown.

Currently, we are conducting a prospective, nonrandomized study to evaluate the feasibility, safety, and effectiveness of a new approach in the treatment of ruptured AAAs. This approach is characterized by the following features: (1) limited fluid resuscitation to prevent rebleed of the aneurysm; (2) routine brachial wire placement under local anesthesia before induction of general anesthesia; (3) deployment of proximal occlusion balloon over this wire for cases with low blood pressure or those that crash after induction; (4) either EVG repair with the VI graft or standard open repair is then carried out, depending on the anatomical characteristics of the aneurysm. This study has already enrolled 12 patients. The preliminary results appear promising, and we have had no patient deaths.

REFERENCES

1. Ernst CB: Abdominal aortic aneurysms. *N Engl J Med* 328:1167-1172, 1993.
2. Wakefield TW, Whitehouse WM, Wu SC: Abdominal aortic aneurysm rupture: Statistical analysis of factors affecting outcome of surgical treatment. *Surgery* 91:586-595, 1982.
3. Donaldson MC, Rosenberg JM, Bucknam CA: Factors affecting survival after ruptured abdominal aortic aneurysm. *J Vasc Surg* 2:564-570, 1985.

4. Shackleton CR, Schechter MT, Bianco R, et al: Preoperative predictors of mortality risk in ruptured abdominal aortic aneurysm. *J Vasc Surg* 6:583-589, 1987.
5. Ouriel K, Geary K, Green RM, et al: Factors determining survival after ruptured aortic aneurysm: The hospital, the surgeon, and the patient. *J Vasc Surg* 11:493-496, 1990.
6. Crawford ES: Ruptured abdominal aortic aneurysm: An editoral. *J Vasc Surg* 13:348-350, 1991.
7. Johansen K, Kohler TR, Nicholls SC, et al: Ruptured abdominal aortic aneurysm: The Harborview experience. *J Vasc Surg* 13:240-247, 1991.
8. Harris LM, Faggioli GL, Fiedler R, et al: Ruptured abdominal aortic aneurysms: Factors affecting mortality rates. *J Vasc Surg* 14:812-820, 1991.
9. Gloviczki P, Pairolero PC, Mucha P: Ruptured abdominal aortic aneurysms: Repair should not be denied. *J Vasc Surg* 15:851-859, 1992.
10. Marty-Ane CH, Alric P, Picot MC, et al: Ruptured abdominal aortic aneurysm: Influence of intraoperative management on surgical outcome. *J Vasc Surg* 22:780-786, 1995.
11. Panneton JM, Lassonde J, Laurendeau F: Ruptured abdominal aortic aneurysm: Impact of comorbidity and postoperative complications on outcome. *Ann Vasc Surg* 9:535-541, 1995.
12. Darling RC, Cordero JA, Chang BB: Advances in the surgical repair of ruptured abdominal aortic aneurysms. *Cardiovasc Surg* 4:720-723, 1996.
13. Farooq MM, Freischlag JA, Seabrook GR, et al: Effect of the duration of symptoms, transport time, and length of emergency room stay on morbidity and mortality in patients with ruptured abdominal aortic aneurysms. *Surgery* 119:9-14, 1996.
14. Lazarides MK, Arvanitis DP, Drista H, et al: POSSUM and APACHE II scores do not predict the outcome of ruptured infrarenal aortic aneurysms. *Ann Vasc Surg* 11:155-158, 1997.
15. Halpern VJ, Kline RG, DiAngelo AJ, et al: Factors that affect the survival rate of patients with ruptured abdominal aortic aneurysms. *J Vasc Surg* 26:939-948, 1997.
16. Dardik A, Burleyson GP, Bowman H, et al: Surgical repair of ruptured abdominal aortic aneurysms in the state of Maryland: Factors influencing outcome among 527 recent cases. *J Vasc Surg* 28:413-421, 1998.
17. Parodi JC, Palmaz JC, Barone HD: Transfemoral intraluminal graft implantation for abdominal aortic aneurysms. *Ann Vasc Surg* 5:491-499, 1991.
18. Blum U, Voshage G, Lammer J, et al: Endoluminal stent-grafts for infrarenal abdominal aortic aneurysms. *N Engl J Med* 336:13-20, 1997.
19. Marin ML, Veith FJ, Cynamon J, et al: Initial experience with transluminally placed endovascular grafts for the treatment of complex vascular lesions. *Ann Surg* 222:1-17, 1995.

20. Ohki T, Marin ML, Veith FJ, et al: Endovascular aorto-uni-iliac grafts and femoro-femoral bypass for bilateral limb threatening ischemia. *J Vasc Surg* 24:984-997, 1996.

21. Marin ML, Veith FJ, Panetta TF, et al: Transluminally placed endovascular stented graft repair for arterial trauma. *J Vasc Surg* 20:466-473, 1994.

22. Ohki T, Marin ML, Veith FJ: Use of endovascular grafts to treat nonaneurysmal arterial disease. *Ann Vasc Surg* 11:200-205, 1997.

23. May J, White GH, Yu W, et al: Concurrent comparison of endoluminal versus open repair in the treatment of abdominal aortic aneurysms: Analysis of 303 patients by life table method. *J Vasc Surg* 29:32-37, 1999.

24. Yusuf SW, Whitaker SC, Chuter TAM, et al: Early results of endovascular aortic aneurysm surgery with aortouniiliac graft, contralateral iliac occlusion, and femorofemoral bypass. *J Vasc Surg* 25:165-172, 1997.

25. Ohki T, Veith FJ, Sanchez LA, et al: Varying strategies and devices for endovascular repair of abdominal aortic aneurysms. *Semin Vasc Surg* 10:242-256, 1997.

26. Yuan JG, Marin ML, Veith FJ, et al: Endovascular grafts for the treatment of para-anastomotic aneurysm. *J Vasc Surg* 26:210-221, 1997.

27. Yusuf SW, Whitaker SC, Chuter TA, et al: Emergency endovascular repair of leaking aortic aneurysm. *Lancet* 344:1645, 1994.

28. Ohki T, Veith FJ: Minimally invasive vascular surgery, in Brooks DC (ed): *Current Review of Minimally Invasive Surgery*, ed 3. Philadelphia, Current Medicine, 1998, pp 125-136.

29. Ohki T, Veith FJ, Sanchez LA, et al: Endovascular graft repair of ruptured aorto-iliac aneurysms. *J Am Coll Surg* 189:102-113, 1999.

30. Zarins CK, White RA, Schwarten D, et al: AneuRx stent graft versus open surgical repair of abdominal aortic aneurysms: Multicenter prospective clinical trial. *J Vasc Surg* 29:292-305, 1999.

CHAPTER 5

Transrenal Fixation of Endovascular Grafts for the Exclusion of Abdominal Aortic Aneurysms

Michael L. Marin, MD
Henry Kaufmann Professor of Vascular Surgery, Mount Sinai School of
Medicine, Director, Endovascular Surgical Development Program, Mount
Sinai Medical Center, New York

Larry H. Hollier, MD
Julius H. Jacobson II, MD, Professor of Vascular Surgery, Mount Sinai
School of Medicine, Chairman, Department of Surgery, Mount Sinai
Medical Center, New York

Endovascular repair of abdominal aortic aneurysms (AAAs) is a
rapidly evolving technique that continues to undergo both procedural and device-related modifications. It was initially apparent to
Parodi et al[1] that few infrarenal aneurysms would be amenable to
simple endovascular repairs with the use of isolated proximal
infrarenal fixation and distal aortic cuff attachment. Although
approximately 85% of aortic aneurysms are in the infrarenal position, on close inspection many of these lesions show insufficient normal aorta immediately below the renal vessels to provide for secure,
long-term attachment of an aortic endograft.[2,3] In 1990, Parodi inserted an endograft with the porous portion of a balloon-expandable
stent attachment system across the orifices of the renal arteries, permitting continued kidney perfusion and successful aortic aneurysm
exclusion in a patient who had a short infrarenal neck (J. C. Parodi,
personal communication, 1990). The feasibility of transrenal endograft attachment and the potential impact on renal perfusion in animal models have been further shown by subsequent laboratory

investigations.[4-11] Early clinical studies have confirmed these findings.[12-15] This chapter reviews the clinical experience with this technique.

TECHNICAL CONCEPT

The placement of aortic endograft attachment systems across the renal artery orifices requires belief in 2 theoretical concepts: (1) that perfusion and function of the renal arteries will not be adversely affected by the positioning of a fenestrated stent within the aorta with possible stent struts across the renal ostia, and (2) that fixation within this "pararenal" aorta will enhance the chances for a durable seal because the pararenal tissue may be stronger and more resistant to radial expansion.

The placement of fenestrated stents across the orifices of arteries is not a new concept. Such positioning has allowed for suc-

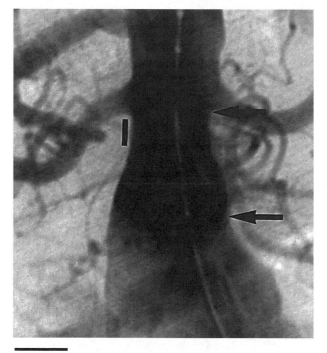

FIGURE 1.

Aortic angiogram demonstrating the anatomy of the "long" infrarenal neck in a patient with an abdominal aortic aneurysm. While on superficial inspection, the aortic neck appears to be quite long *(distance between the arrows)*, a closer look identifies a "ring" of normal tissue just below the renal arteries *(solid bar)* with the remaining "neck" showing an irregular (plaque containing) surface with a tendency toward enlargement.

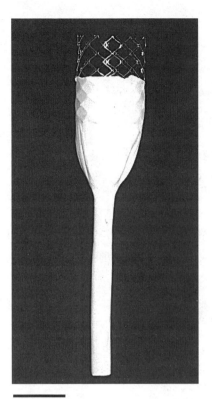

FIGURE 2.
Photograph of a Parodi-Palmaz aortoiliac stent graft device, fabricated from a stainless steel balloon expandable stent and a tapered expanded polytetrafluoroethylene (ePTFE) graft. The stent, seen in the deployed state, is fixed to the graft material by 4 "U" stitches.

cessful stent placement and normal vessel perfusion in both peripheral vascular and coronary circulation.[16,17] Furthermore, subsequent interventions within the "jailed" side branch may be performed using standard catheter-based techniques, including angioplasty and stenting. The successful placement of metallic stents within the orifices of the renal arteries for the treatment of renal artery occlusive disease further suggests the relative safety of pararenal stent positioning.[18]

The second concept of enhanced pararenal tissue integrity is somewhat more speculative. It has been observed that the 1-cm segment of aortic tissue immediately below the lowest renal artery is more likely to be free of ectatic changes or aneurysmal degeneration than the caudad region of the vessels. This is also notable in patients who have a seemingly long (>2 cm) aortic neck (Fig 1).

Whether this segment of the artery will provide a more durable seal, free from late dilatation, awaits further follow-up.

METHODS AND DEVICES

Virtually all aortic endografts that have an open or fenestrated proximal stent attachment device have been used for transrenal fixation. Superiority of individual devices has not been determined.

BALLOON-EXPANDABLE PARODI-PALMAZ SYSTEM

At our institution, we have had extensive experience with the balloon expandable Parodi-Palmaz system for treating patients with short pararenal necks.

The transrenal attachment system is created from a Palmaz balloon expandable stent (P5014, Cordis Endovascular, Johnson & Johnson, Warren, NJ) and a 28- to 8-mm tapered expanded polyte-

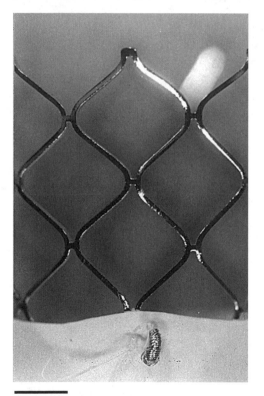

FIGURE 3.
High magnification photograph of the expanded Parodi-Palmaz attachment system. The typical space between struts is 6.3 × 6.0 mm. Each strut is approximately 0.3 mm thick.

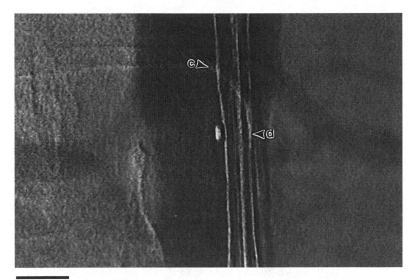

FIGURE 4.
Intraoperative angiogram demonstrating the use of a diagnostic catheter *(c)* inserted through the contralateral common femoral artery for dynamic imaging during transrenal endograft placement. The position of the endograft within its delivery catheter *(a)* is adjusted to reside at the base of the lowest renal artery.

trafluoroethylene (ePTFE) graft (8-mm thin-walled graft, Impra, Tempe, Ariz) (Fig 2). At an example expansion of 26 mm, the fenestrated portions of the stent measured 6.3 × 6.0 mm, with a stent thickness of 0.3 mm (Fig 3).

Each stent is fixed to the tapered ePTFE graft by means of 4 ePTFE sutures (CV5, W.L. Gore and Associates, Flagstaff, Ariz). When the endograft is deployed to 26 mm, 20 mm of uncovered stent projects from the undeployed device; expected foreshortening of the stent results in 12 mm of bare stent for transrenal fixation. The total transrenal segment varies between 11 and 13 mm. For precise positioning, a gold marker is placed at the interface between the graft and the underlying stent to mark the site where the graft begins. Each endovascular graft is coaxially attached to a customized balloon catheter delivery system and gas sterilized before use (Fig 4).

Technique for Endovascular Graft Insertion With the Use of the Parodi-Palmaz System

Endovascular grafts contained within a delivery catheter are advanced over a 0.038-inch Amplatz super stiff wire to the pararenal segment of the aorta. A diagnostic catheter is positioned in a similar location within the aorta through the opposite common femoral artery. This diagnostic catheter permits dynamic angiography for precise device positioning (Fig 4). The delivery catheter containing the endograft is retracted caudally, and the endovascular graft is finally positioned before deployment within the aorta so the gold marker on the graft margin is aligned with the inferior border of the lowest renal artery. This position allows the open portion of the stent to extend across the orifices of both renal arteries. To ensure that downward migration of the graft does not occur during balloon deployment, each patient is given 24 mg of adenosine to induce a short (7-10 second) period of asystole before balloon inflation and stent deployment.[19] During this asys-

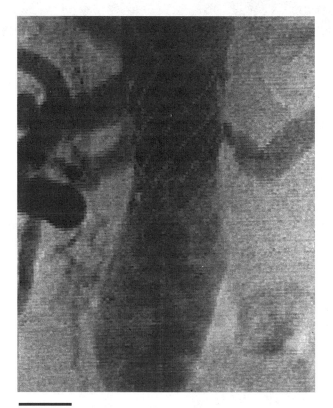

FIGURE 5.
Intraoperative angiogram after balloon-expandable stent deployment. The entire graft portion of the endograft lies below the renal artery ostia, while the fenestrated (open) part of the stent permits free flow of blood into the kidneys.

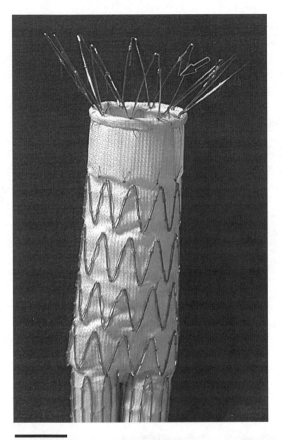

FIGURE 6.
The Cook-Zenith aortic endograft. A thin-walled polyester graft is supported by "Z" shaped stainless steel stents to form a modular endograft. The transrenal attachment system contains barbs fixed to the apices of the cephalad end of the stent *(arrow)*.

tolic period, deployment balloon inflation fixes the endograft to the aortic wall with the entire uncovered (porous) portion of the stent positioned across the renal arteries (Fig 5). (For additional details, see Marin et al[15]) The experience using this system showed a significant reduction in proximal aortic endograft leaks in patients with short necks compared with similar patients in whom the device was placed completely infrarenal ($P \leq .05$).[15] There was no change in serum creatinine level or luminal patency after stent graft placement transrenally. Follow-up extends to 3 years.

COOK-ZENITH STENT GRAFT SYSTEM

The Cook-Zenith stent graft system (Cook, Inc, Bloomington, Ind) is based on the Gianturco "Z" stent design and includes a modular bifurcated construction. Each "Z" stent is composed of stainless steel material. Thin-walled polyester graft material lines the prosthesis (Fig 6). These barbed elements are fixed to the proximal portion of the transrenal attachment system to achieve tight fixation.

TALENT TRANSRENAL SYSTEM

One of the first commercially available transrenal systems was the Talent Device (World Medical Co, Fort Lauderdale, Fla). The endo-

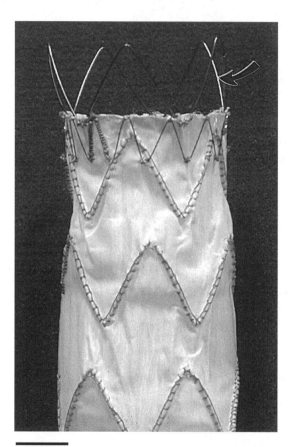

FIGURE 7.
Photograph of the Talent transrenal aortic endograft system. "Z" shaped nitinol wire stents are fully sutured onto the graft wall to provide structural support. "Z" configured nitinol devoid of graft material extends across the renal orifices to achieve transrenal fixation *(arrow)*.

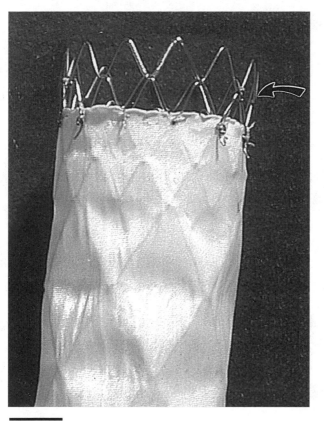

FIGURE 8.
Photograph of the Vanguard aortic endograft. The cephalad 1 cm of the aortic attachment system is uncovered for possible transrenal placement *(arrow).*

graft is constructed from "Z" configured nitinol stents, which are completely sutured to a seamed, thin-walled polyester vascular graft (Fig 7). Specified figure-of-eight markers at the stent-to-graft interface assist in proper placement of this device in the transrenal position. The Talent endograft is used in tubular and modular bifurcated configurations.

VANGUARD AORTIC ENDOGRAFT
The Vanguard aortic endograft (Boston Scientific Co, Natick, Mass) is constructed of "Z" configured nitinol metal stents sutured to one another and to a thin-walled polyester graft by polypropylene sutures. One centimeter of the proximal stent is uncovered and has thus been used for transrenal placement (Fig 8).[13] The specified

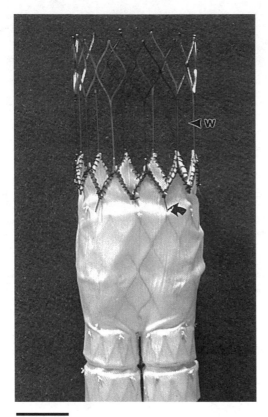

FIGURE 9.
Photograph of the Ariba transrenal aortic endograft (Teramed). This device contains a transrenal attachment system with open spaces ("windows") to allow unobstructed renal perfusion *(w)*. Fixation barbs are located below the renal ostia to ensure tight aortic fixation *(arrow)*. The modular design permits ipsilateral and contralateral iliac limb length adjustment after the device has been inserted into the body.

"V" shaped marker at the upper graft margin assists in proper alignment.

ARIBA AORTIC ENDOGRAFT

The Ariba aortic endograft (Teramed, Minneapolis, Minn) has been specifically designed to permit transrenal placement. The transrenal attachment system has wide "windows" that bridge across the renal ostia (Fig 9). Self-deploying barbs are designed to engage the aorta within the "preserved" 1-cm aortic ring below the lowest renal artery. This permits a function seal suprarenally and a barb-penetration seal below the renal arteries. The stent support components of the

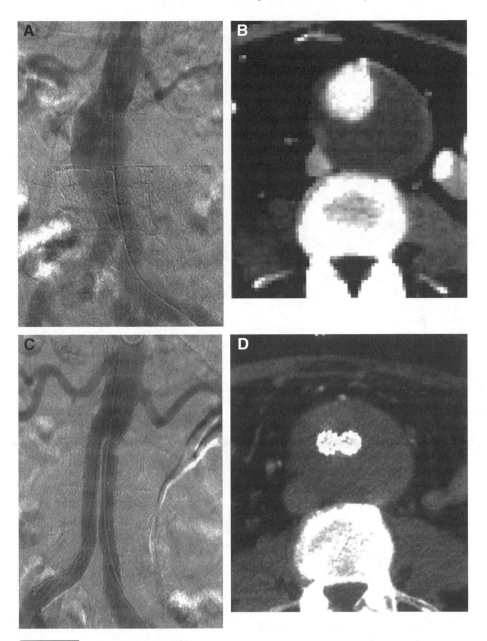

FIGURE 10.
Endovascular repair of an abdominal aortic aneurysm (AAA) with the Teramed Ariba device using transrenal fixation. **A,** Preoperative aortogram demonstrating an infrarenal AAA. **B,** Computed tomography (CT) scan of the abdomen identifies
(continued)

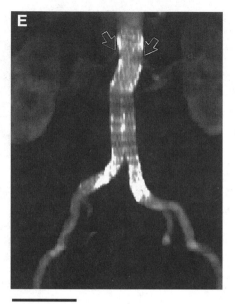

FIGURE 10. (continued)
a thrombus-filled AAA measuring 6.0 cm. **C,** Angiogram of the AAA after insertion of the Ariba device. Each iliac limb length has been adjusted "in situ" to allow the endograft to extend to the takeoff of the internal iliac artery. The AAA no longer opacifies. **D,** CT scan after AAA exclusion with the Ariba endovascular graft device. Contrast is confined to iliac graft lumens indicating aneurysm exclusion. **E,** CT scan demonstrating the maximum intensity projection after AAA exclusion. The transrenal segment can be identified along with the right and left renal arteries projecting through the stent *(arrows).*

endograft are covered with a thin-walled seamless polyester graft. Clinical trials of this graft in Europe have shown favorable early results (Fig 10).

SUMMARY

The durability of endovascular repair of abdominal aortic aneurysms depends largely on creating and maintaining a long-term seal between the pararenal aorta and the aortic endograft. The likelihood of achieving this may be enhanced by transrenal graft fixation, particularly in patients who have a short region of normal aorta below the renal vessels. Long-term follow-up will be needed to ensure preservation of normal renal function.

REFERENCES

1. Parodi JC, Palmaz JC, Barone HD: Transfemoral intraluminal graft implantation for abdominal aortic aneurysms. *Ann Vasc Surg* 5:491-499, 1991.

2. Schumacher H, Eckstein HH, Kallinowski F, et al: Morphometry and classification in abdominal aortic aneurysms: Patient selection for endovascular and open surgery. *J Endovasc Surg* 4:39-44, 1997.
3. Illig KA, Green RM, Ouriel K, et al: Fate of the proximal aortic cuff: Implications for endovascular aneurysm repair. *J Vasc Surg* 26:492-501, 1997.
4. Malina M, Lindh M, Ivancev K, et al: The effects of endovascular aortic stents placed across the renal arteries. *Eur J Vasc Endovasc Surg* 13:207-213, 1997.
5. Whitbread T, Birch P, Rogers S, et al: The effect of placing an aortic wall stent across thc renal artery origins in an animal model. *Eur J Vasc Endovasc Surg* 13:154-158, 1997.
6. Lawrence DO, Charnsangave C, Wright KC, et al: Percutaneous endovascular graft: Experimental evaluation. *Radiology* 163:357-360, 1987.
7. Mirich D, Wright KC, Wallace S, et al: Percutaneously placed endovascular grafts for aortic aneurysms: Feasibility study. *Radiology* 170:1033-1037, 1989.
8. Nasim A, Thompson MM, Sayers T, et al: Investigation of the relationship between aortic stent position and renal function. *J Endovasc Surg* 2:90-91, 1995.
9. Ruiz CE, Zhang HP, Douglas JT: A novel method for treatment of abdominal aortic aneurysms using percutaneous implantation of a newly designed endovascular device. *Circulation* 91:2470-2477, 1995.
10. Ferko A, Krajina A, Jon B, et al: Juxtarenal aortic aneurysms: Endoluminal transfemoral repair? *Eur Radiol* 7:703-707, 1997.
11. Desgranges P, Hutin E, Kedzia C, et al: Aortic stents covering the renal artery ostia: An animal study. *J Vasc Intervent Radiol* 8:77-82, 1997.
12. Lawrence-Brown M, Hartley D, MacSweeney ST, et al: The Perth endoluminal bifurcated graft system: Development and early experience. *Cardiovasc Surg* 4:706-712, 1996.
13. Duda SH, Raygrotzki S, Wisklrchen J, et al: Abdominal aortic aneurysms: Treatment with juxtarenal placement of covered stent grafts. *Radiology* 206-209, 1998.
14. Malina M, Brunkwall K, Ivancev K, et al: Renal arteries covered by aortic stents: Clinical experience from endovascular grafting of aortic aneurysms. *Eur J Endovasc Surg* 14:109-113, 1997.
15. Marin ML, Parsons RE, Hollier LH, et al: Impact of transrenal aortic endograft placement on endovascular graft repair of abdominal aortic aneurysms. *J Vasc Surg* 28:638-646, 1998.
16. Pan M, Medina A, Hernandez E, et al: Follow-up patency of side branches covered by an intracoronary Palmaz-Schatz stent. *Circulation* 88:I-640, 1993.
17. Long AL, Page PE, Raynaud AC, et al: Percutaneous iliac artery stent: Angiographic long-term follow-up. *Radiology* 180:771-778, 1991.

18. Blum U, Krumme B, Frugel P, et al: Treatment of ostial renal-artery stenosis with vascular endoprostheses often unsuccessful balloon angioplasty. *N Eng J Med* 336:459-495, 1997.
19. Dorms G, Cohn JM: Adenosine-induced transient cardiac asystole enhances precise deployment of stent-grafts in the thoracic and abdominal aorta. *J Endovasc Surg* 3:275-278, 1996.

PART III

Infrainguinal Disease

CHAPTER 6

Duplex-monitored Angioplasty of Peripheral Artery and Infrainguinal Vein Graft Stenosis

Brad L. Johnson, MD
Assistant Professor of Surgery, Division of Vascular Surgery, University of South Florida College of Medicine, Tampa

Anthony J. Avino, MD
Fellow, Division of Vascular Surgery, University of South Florida College of Medicine, Tampa

Dennis F. Bandyk, MD
Professor of Surgery, Division of Vascular Surgery, University of South Florida College of Medicine, Tampa

The endovascular treatment of infrainguinal arterial occlusive disease, although widely practiced, has been viewed with some skepticism by vascular surgeons. Since the introduction of transluminal artery dilation by Dotter in 1964, percutaneous transluminal angioplasty (PTA) of occlusive lesions involving the femoropopliteal arterial segment has been associated with inferior patency rates when compared with infrainguinal vein bypass. A major problem has been the unpredictable durability of the procedure. Early failure rates from 9% to 47% after PTA have been reported, with modes of failure such as elastic recoil at the PTA site, plaque dissection, and spasm complicated by thrombus formation implicated.[1-3] The frequency of technical failure has correlated with type of lesion (occlusion vs stenosis), status of runoff arteries (diffuse vs focal atherosclerotic disease), and severity of limb ischemia (tissue loss vs claudication).[3] Thus, treatment of an occluded artery segment in a limb with digit gangrene and diffuse popliteal-tibial artery atherosclerosis would be associated with the highest early failure rate. Attempts to improve the outcome of femoropopliteal PTA with the use of adjunctive measures of prolonged balloon inflation time or stent placement have not significantly enhanced results. An important question that needs to be addressed is whether arterio-graphy alone is a valid method to judge the technical success of a PTA procedure. We believe duplex ultrasonography may be a more appropriate diagnostic technique to evaluate peripheral angioplasty sites for residual stenosis.

Although intravascular ultrasound (IVUS) and the measurement of systolic pressure gradient across an arterial stenosis can yield useful end point criteria during PTA, their application is better suited for monitoring aortoiliac endovascular procedures. By comparison, duplex scanning is ideally suited for imaging the arterial tree below the inguinal ligament and identifying sites of stenosis.[4] Several vascular centers that have used duplex ultrasonography to evaluate the hemodynamics of PTA sites confirm a significant incidence of residual stenosis despite an angiogram showing less than 30% diameter reduction (DR) residual stenosis.[1,5] Although a high diagnostic accuracy for duplex scanning in grading carotid artery disease severity or assessing the outcome of carotid endarterectomy is accepted clinically, the application of peripheral duplex testing to monitor the outcome of endovascular procedures has not been encouraged. Mewissen et al[1] demonstrated that approximately one quarter of femoropopliteal PTA sites without residual stenosis by arteriography had abnormal velocity spectra, indicating greater than 50% DR stenosis when examined with color duplex scanning. The finding of a residual PTA stenosis by duplex scanning was predictive of clinical deterioration and PTA failure. By life-table analysis, a greater than 50% DR PTA site residual stenosis by duplex-derived velocity spectra criteria (peak systolic velocity [PSV] > 180 cm/s; velocity ratio [Vr] at site > 2.5) was associated with a 1-year clinical success rate of only 15% versus an 84% stenosis-free patency when a less than 50% DR residual stenosis was verified. Spikjkerboer et al[5] also reported that a residual duplex stenosis 1 day after PTA was prognostic for failure within 1 year. These observations provide the basis for the application of duplex surveillance during or immediately after PTA to verify the technical adequacy of the procedure.

SELECTION OF STENOSIS FOR PTA

The proper selection of patients with infrainguinal arterial or vein graft stenosis for endovascular treatment significantly affects both

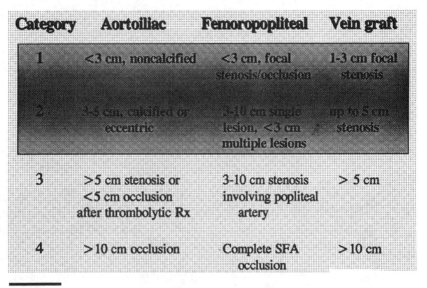

Category	Aortoiliac	Femoropopliteal	Vein graft
1	<3 cm, noncalcified	<3 cm, focal stenosis/occlusion	1-3 cm focal stenosis
2	3-5 cm, calcified or eccentric	3-10 cm single lesion, <3 cm multiple lesions	up to 5 cm stenosis
3	>5 cm stenosis or <5 cm occlusion after thrombolytic Rx	3-10 cm stenosis involving popliteal artery	> 5 cm
4	>10 cm occlusion	Complete SFA occlusion	>10 cm

FIGURE 1.
Society of Cardiovascular and Interventional Radiology *(SCVIR)* classification of arterial lesions for suitability of treatment by percutaneous transluminal angioplasty *(PTA). Abbreviation: SFA,* Superior femoral artery.

the initial and the long-term success of the intervention. Patients with symptomatic peripheral arterial disease should undergo a clinical evaluation (history, physical examination, assessment of atherosclerotic risk factors and comorbid conditions) and vascular laboratory evaluation, including duplex mapping of the arterial system. On the basis of duplex findings, patients found to have unilateral focal stenosis or short (<10 cm) occlusions of recent onset (< 3 months) involving the common iliac or superficial femoral arteries can be considered for PTA (balloon angioplasty/stent with or without catheter-directed thrombolysis). The common femoral artery should be free of significant disease, and the site of angioplasty should not have aneurysmal dilatation. Anatomical features of the arterial lesion and adjacent artery segment should be verified by means of angiography and, if judged to be a category 1 or 2 lesion (based on the Society of Cardiovascular and Interventional Radiology guidelines[6]) endovascular intervention should be performed (Fig 1). A number of classification schemes based on peak systolic velocity (PSV) and PSV ratio across the stenosis have been validated compared with contrast arteriography and are useful in grading stenosis from minor to high grade. In general, a significant flow-reducing stenosis (ie, associated with >20 mm Hg resting systolic pressure gradient) is accurately predicted by duplex scanning when the following findings are present:

1. Loss of the normal triphasic waveform configuration distal to the stenosis.
2. PSV is greater than 300 cm/s.
3. End-diastolic velocity is greater than 20 cm/s.
4. PSV ratio across the stenosis is greater than 3.
5. Distal velocity waveform is damped (decrease in systolic acceleration time).

In our laboratory, a peripheral artery lesion is graded as greater than 75% diameter reducing when the PSV is greater than 300 cm/s, end-diastolic velocity is greater than 100 cm/s, and the PSV ratio is greater than 4.

Endovascular treatment of these categories of lesions is associated with high (95%) technical success rates and clinical outcomes similar to those after bypass grafting. Vessel patency and hemodynamic improvement at 2 years is approximately 80%. By comparison, category 3 lesions (>4-cm length calcific stenosis, multilevel disease, 5- to 10-cm length chronic occlusions), although also amenable to PTA, are associated with higher failure rates with endovascular intervention compared with bypass grafting. PTA of these lesions should only be considered for patients with severe cardiac disease and critical ischemia, patients with unfavorable anatomy for bypass grafts, or patients with no autologous vein for use as a bypass conduit.

Preintervention duplex scanning should minimize the following scenario: an arteriogram is performed, but the referring vascular surgeon is unavailable to review and discuss the findings with the interventional radiologist. An unplanned or inappropriate PTA is performed, or the patient is rescheduled for PTA at a second angiographic session. In a review of 110 patients who underwent lower limb duplex scanning before arteriography at the University of Washington Vascular Laboratory, 50 arterial lesions were considered suitable for PTA based on duplex findings.[7] Of these, PTA was actually carried out in 47 (94%). In the remaining 3 cases, the lesions were verified by arteriography, but technical factors precluded PTA. Importantly, no angioplasties were performed in patients found not to be candidates by duplex scanning.

Duplex scanning also has a proven application for surveillance after infrainguinal bypass grafting and hemodialysis graft placement. Serial studies permit identification of graft stenosis, usually in asymptomatic patients. When left untreated, most bypasses will thrombose. We have observed that early appearing (<3 months) or residual vein graft or anastomotic stenoses are not suited for PTA, as are diffuse vein graft stenoses or focal lesions in small-diameter (<3 mm) vein conduits. Clinical and duplex features of graft lesions best suited for PTA are as follows:

1. Slowly progressive lesions of myointimal hyperplasia or atherosclerotic disease more than 6 months after the primary procedure.
2. PSV greater than 300 cm/s, and Vr across stenosis greater than 3.5.
3. Focal stenosis (<2 cm in length).
4. Vein diameter greater than 3.5 mm.
5. Stenosis involving outflow artery without diffuse atherosclerosis.

When arteriography verified a concentric focal stenosis in an otherwise normal vein bypass, PTA of the lesion resulted in stenosis-free patency of 63% at 2 years, identical to surgical repair of more extensive or early appearing bypass graft stenosis.[8] In our experience, approximately two thirds of vein graft lesions judged to require repair can undergo either surgical or endovascular intervention based on duplex scan findings alone.

DUPLEX-MONITORED ANGIOPLASTY

In treating femoropopliteal arterial segment or infrainguinal vein bypass graft stenosis with endovascular techniques, a number of vascular groups have found the use of angiographic criteria to guide technical success to be misleading.[9-12] Although IVUS is an accurate method to assess PTA site anatomy, transcutaneous duplex ultrasonography can yield similar information, is more cost-effective, and provides data on flow hemodynamics. The velocity spectra recorded proximal to, at the site of angioplasty, and distally, have been found to be more accurate than arteriography in assessing technical success. In approximately 20% of peripheral PTA procedures when arteriography has indicated successful dilatation based on a less than 30% residual stenosis, a duplex scan has indicated residual stenosis based on PSV at the angioplasty site of greater than 180 cm/s and Vr greater than 2. We have used these criteria based on our prior experience of duplex surveillance after femoropopliteal PTA.[1]

The goal of duplex-monitored angioplasty is to ensure that both the angiographic result and the duplex assessment of PTA site hemodynamics are normalized. Prior PTA duplex scanning should evaluate the velocities proximal, at the lesion, and distal to it (Fig 2). After intervention, the treated artery or vein bypass segment is initially assessed with angiography (Fig 3). If a greater than 30% DR residual stenosis is demonstrated, the lesions should be further dilated. When no residual stenosis is confirmed by arteriography, the treated segment should be imaged by color Doppler and velocity spectra recordings obtained identical to the pre-PTA study. The pre-PTA velocity spectra would typically indicate high-grade, pressure-reducing stenosis with a PSV greater than 300 cm/s and an end-diastolic velocity greater than 40 cm/s. After successful PTA, the PSV at the site of stenosis and/or angioplasty should be

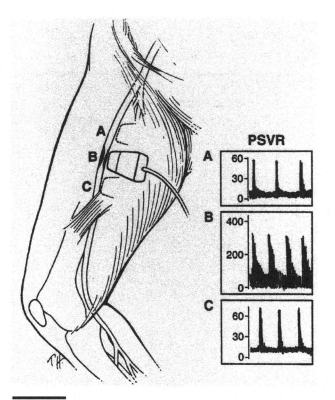

FIGURE 2.
Schematic of transcutanous duplex scanning during peripheral angioplasty procedure. The site of stenosis is imaged before, during, and after endovascular intervention. Classification of residual stenosis is based on changes in peak systolic velocity *(PSV)* recorded across the lesions with calculation of a PSV ratio *(PSVR)*. A PSVR value greater than 2 indicates a significant residual stenosis when associated with a PSV greater than 180 cm/s.

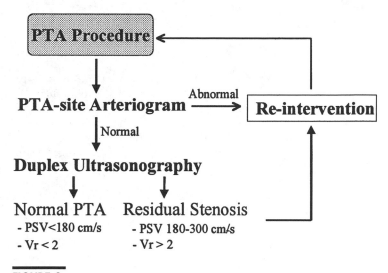

FIGURE 3.
Evaluation algorithm of peripheral percutaneous transluminal angioplasty *(PTA)* using arteriography and duplex ultrasonography.
Abbreviation: Vr, Velocity ratio.

less than 180 cm/s, and the Vr across the treated stenotic segment should be less than 2.

In the treatment of 18 atherosclerotic stenoses involving the femoropopliteal arterial segment and 30 infrainguinal vein graft stenoses, duplex scanning performed during the PTA procedure altered treatment in 12 instances (Table 1). The finding of a residual stenosis based on velocity spectra criteria led to use of a longer balloon in 7 cases, a longer inflation time (>3 minutes) in 3 cases, and placement of a stent in 2 cases. Overall, stenosis-free patency was 78% at 2 years, an outcome similar to our results of infrainguinal bypass grafting for symptomatic femoropopliteal atherosclerotic occlusive disease or surgical intervention for vein graft stenosis.

The following cases illustrate angiographic and duplex findings in typical cases of duplex-monitored angioplasty.

Case 1. A 67-year-old woman had a redo femoral-popliteal bypass using cephalic vein for ischemic rest pain. Postoperative graft surveillance 6 months later identified a greater than 80% DR focal stenosis with velocity spectra (PSV = 410 cm/s) that met our criteria for treatment by PTA (Fig 4). Despite a normal-appearing angiographic result after PTA with a 6-mm × 4-cm balloon, duplex scanning revealed a greater than 50% DR residual stenosis (PSV = 205 cm/s). A repeat PTA using a 7-mm × 4-cm balloon normalized velocity spectra at the PTA with a decrease in PSV to 84 cm/s.

Case 2. A 73-year-old man had undergone a femoral to anterior tibial saphenous vein bypass that developed a focal 80% DR stenosis at the distal anastomosis. After PTA with a 3-mm balloon, duplex assessment of the site identified a persistent elevation in PSV to 229 cm/s (Vr ≥ 2.8) despite an angiogram showing no residual stenosis (Fig 5). Repeat PTA with a larger 4-mm balloon produced a reduction in PSV to 102 cm/s.

When a lesion is judged to be maximally dilated but duplex scanning detects a persistent stenosis, further PTA risks artery or vein bypass rupture and should be avoided. Other endovascular options to be considered include atherectomy or stent deployment. In the case of an infrainguinal vein graft stenosis, either continued surveillance or operative intervention of the residual stenosis is an appropriate treatment option, depending on the severity of the stenosis. A persistent duplex-detected stenosis at the angioplasty site has, in our experience, correlated with early failure by progression to stenosis with similar hemodynamics as the primary lesion, or to occlusion. In treating infrainguinal vein graft stenosis, we prefer to proceed with surgical repair when PSV at the PTA site exceeds 200 cm/s and the Vr at the site is greater than 2.5.

The use of intraoperative duplex scanning to verify a normal hemodynamic result after arterial surgery has been associated with a low incidence of early failure and late restenosis. After carotid endarterectomy, we have observed a reduction in recurrent stenosis involving either the internal or common carotid artery from approximately 15% to less than 5% with routine intraoperative

TABLE 1.

University of South Florida Experience With Duplex-monitored PTA of Femoropopliteal Arterial Stenosis or Infrainguinal Vein Graft Stenosis

Site of PTA	No. of Sites	Treatment Altered*	Early Failure	Late Failure
Femoropopliteal stenosis	18	4	0	1
Vein graft stenosis	30	8	1	4†

*Larger balloon (n = 7); longer inflation time (n = 3); stent placement (n = 2).
†80% stenosis-free patency at 2 years.
Abbreviation: PTA, Percutaneous transluminal balloon angioplasty.

PSV = 410 cm/s   PSV = 205 cm/s   PSV = 84 cm/s

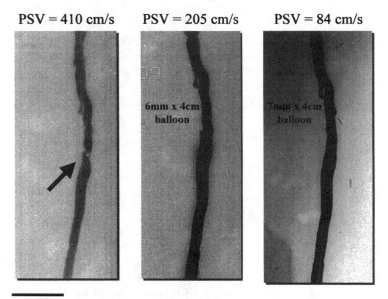

FIGURE 4.
Angiograms and peak systolic velocity *(PSV)* measurements obtained before and after balloon angioplasty of an infrainguinal vein graft stenosis.

assessment by duplex ultrasound. On the basis of this experience, we expanded the application of duplex scanning to assess the technical adequacy of a variety of arterial interventions including infrainguinal bypass, renal visceral bypass, and femoropopliteal vein bypass PTA.

Duplex monitoring of the PTA procedure has been most rewarding in the treatment of infrainguinal vein graft stenosis. We have verified that balloon angioplasty of a focal stenosis can normalize velocity spectra within the treated graft segment (Fig 6). In a consecutive series of 30 infrainguinal vein graft PTAs, PSV of the stenosis decreased from 408 ± 126 cm/s (range, 300-540 cm/s) to 126 ± 42 cm/s (range, 85-220 cm/s). In 12 PTA procedures, duplex imaging performed after a satisfactory angiographic resolution of stenosis was achieved showed that the PSV in the treated site was greater than 180 cm/s (mean, 253 cm/s). After reintervention, the mean PSV decreased to 126 cm/s. In only one instance did the PSV remain greater than 180 cm/s. We believe the addition of duplex monitoring can enhance the outcome of PTA procedures by verifying whether hemodynamics are normal or a residual stenosis remains. In 38 vein graft stenoses treated by PTA without duplex monitoring, the velocity spectra recording after PTA indicated a higher incidence of residual stenosis (PSV = 164 ± 74 cm/s). A PSV greater than 180 cm/s was recorded in 6 of the treated graft segments.

Does normalization of PTA site velocity spectra improve durability of the procedure? In our experience, it does. The stenosis-free patency at 1-year was 89% after duplex-monitored PTA compared with 61% for PTA without duplex assessment ($P < .05$, log rank). Katzenschlager et al[12] of the University of Vienna confirmed that the results of PTA with duplex ultrasound guidance for treatment of short stenoses or occlusions in the superficial femoral or popliteal artery were similar to the results achieved with PTA performed under fluoroscopic control. In 3 of 25 successful PTAs, duplex ultrasound indicated residual stenosis and PTA with a larger balloon was repeated. Duplex monitoring has also been used with an ultrasound-guided catheter system that permits PTA without ionizing radiation and relies on duplex-detected changes in hemodynamic parameters during angioplasty to verify successful dilation. The criteria for success was a Vr of less than 2.0 across the treated artery segment. In a report by Cluley et al,[10] supplemental use of a high-pressure ballon or an atherectomy device was necessary in 5 (29%) of 17 patients because of a residual duplex-identified abnormality.

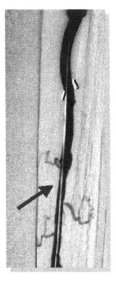

PTA 3mm balloon: PSV = 229 cm/s

PTA 4mm balloon: PSV = 102 cm/s

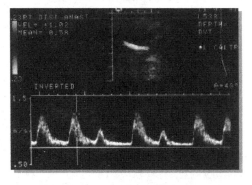

PSV = 102 cm/s

FIGURE 5.
Angiogram and duplex-derived velocity spectra recorded during balloon angioplasty of an anastomotic stenosis. *Abbreviations: PTA,* Percutaneous transluminal angioplasty; *PSV,* peak systolic velocity.

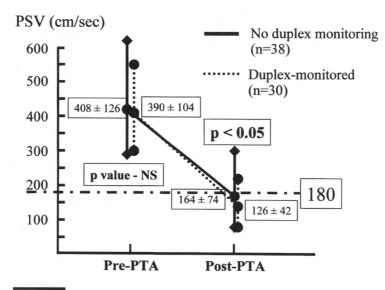

FIGURE 6.
Peak systolic velocity *(PSV)* measurements obtained before and after percutaneous transluminal angioplasty *(PTA)* in the treatment of infrainguinal vein grafts with and without duplex monitoring.

FOLLOW-UP RECOMMENDATIONS

Late failure of PTA can result from restenosis within the treated
segment most commonly caused by the development of myointimal hyperplasia, or from progression of atherosclerosis at and
remote from the PTA site. Occasionally, a combination of both disease processes results in a recurrence of limb ischemia symptoms.
Identification of a failing PTA does not preclude redilation, stent
placement, or both, and a repeat PTA is generally associated with
a prognosis identical to that of the primary procedure.

Lower limb PTA procedures should be assessed by duplex scanning and measurement of the ankle-brachial index (ABI). If duplex
monitoring during the procedure is performed and no residual
stenosis is detected, we perform a follow-up duplex assessment in
approximately 1 to 2 weeks. If duplex scanning documents a residual stenosis, the study should be repeated the next day. This is
usually feasible because most patients are admitted on a 23-hour
outpatient basis. If a normal PTA site is confirmed by duplex testing (ie, <50% DR residual stenosis, ABI > 0.2 compared with pre-
PTA level), follow-up surveillance at 3 months and then every 6
months thereafter is recommended. If the postprocedure duplex
scan identifies a 50% to 75% DR stenosis but ABI has increased

appropriately, serial scans at 4- to 6-week intervals should be performed to evaluate for functional deterioration at the PTA site. A progressive PTA site stenosis should be subjected to repeat dilation, atherectomy, or stent placement, depending on the anatomical characteristics of the lesion and arterial segment.

COST-EFFECTIVENESS

No reported study has verified the cost-benefit aspects of duplex monitoring during and after PTA. Assumptions that PTA is less expensive therapy compared with surgical bypass grafting have proved to be correct, particularly when the efficacy of PTA is based on strict outcome criteria and reporting standards. A recent report indicated the ratio of hospital costs of PTA to bypass surgery was 53% for patients treated for claudication but increased to 75% for those with critical ischemia.[3] Angioplasty failure is expensive, and efforts to improve the durability of these procedures must be encouraged. Tielbeek et al[9] found that although duplex surveillance can identify PTA site restenosis, clinical and hemodynamic criteria were more useful in selecting patients for reintervention. The predictive value of duplex-monitored PTA needs to be further documented, but it does appear that a PTA site with normal arterial hemodynamics as assessed by color duplex ultrasonography is associated with a durability comparable to saphenous vein bypass grafting. Because PTA has a failure incidence similar to infrainguinal vein bypass, the cost-effectiveness and efficacy of surveillance should be comparable. Whether duplex surveillance can identify those patients who would benefit from a redo endovascular procedure is not known.

SUMMARY

Similar to standard surgical arterial interventions, the outcome of endovascular procedures must be continually analyzed to ensure optimal results. By providing hemodynamic information, duplex ultrasonography has lessened the need for invasive angiograms to assess results, and when used during intervention, duplex ultrasonography can improve technical precision by reducing the frequency of residual stenosis. Surveillance studies conducted to date uniformly indicate a higher failure rate for the hemodynamically flawed arterial repair. Our preliminary results using duplex-monitored angioplasty demonstrated a significant yield with intraprocedural testing. In approximately one fourth of cases, a residual stenosis is detected and further endovascular therapy can normalize flow hemodynamics. Duplex-monitored angioplasty applied to the appropriately selected artery or vein graft stenosis allows a less-invasive intervention and attempts to optimize the benefit of endovascular treatment of lower limb occlusive disease.

REFERENCES

1. Mewissen MW, Kinney EV, Bandyk DF, et al: The role of duplex scanning versus angiography in predicting outcome after balloon angioplasty in the femoropopliteal artery. *J Vasc Surg* 15:860-864, 1992.
2. Hunik MGM, Wong JB, Donaldson MC, et al: Patency results of percutaneous and surgical femoropopliteal revascularization procedures. *Med Decis Making* 14:71-81, 1994.
3. Hunink MGM, Cullen KA, Donaldson MC: Hospital costs of revascularization procedures for femoropopliteal arterial disease. *J Vasc Surg* 19:632-641, 1994.
4. Van der Heijden FH, Legemote DA, Leeuwen MS, et al: Value of duplex scanning in the selection of patients for percutaneous transluminal angioplasty. *Eur J Vasc Surg* 7:71-76, 1993.
5. Spijkerboer AM, Nass PC, de Valois JC, et al: Evaluation of femoropopliteal arteries with duplex ultrasound after angioplasty. Can we predict results at one year? *Eur J Vasc Endovasc Surg* 12:418-423, 1996.
6. Standards of Practice Committee of the Society of Cardiovascular and Interventional Radiology: Guidelines for percutaneous angioplasty. *Radiology* 177:619-630, 1990.
7. Edwards JM, Coldwell DM, Goldman ML, et al: The role of duplex scanning in the selection of patients for transluminal angioplasty. *J Vasc Surg* 13:69-74, 1991.
8. Avino AJ, Bandyk DF, Gonsalves AJ, et al: Surgical and endovascular intervention for infrainguinal vein graft stenosis. *J Vasc Surg* 29:60-71, 1999.
9. Tielbeek AV, Rietjens E, Buth J, et al: The value of duplex surveillance after endovascular intervention for femoropopliteal obstructive disease. *Eur J Vasc Endovasc Surg* 12:145-150, 1996.
10. Cluley SR, Brener BJ, Hollier L, et al: Transcutaneous ultrasonography can be used to guide and monitor balloon angioplasty. *J Vasc Surg* 17:23-31, 1993.
11. Ramaswami G, Al-kutoubi A, Nicolaides AN, et al: Duplex controlled angioplasty. *Eur J Vasc Surg* 8:457-463, 1994.
12. Katzenschlager R, Ahmadi A, Minar E, et al: Femoropopliteal artery: Initial and 6-month results of color duplex US-guided percutaneous transluminal angioplasty. *Radiology* 199:331-334, 1996.

CHAPTER 7

Functional Outcome of Surgery for Limb Salvage

Alexander D. Nicoloff, MD
Fellow, Division of Vascular Surgery, Oregon Health Sciences University,
Portland

Ahmed M. Abou-Zamzam, Jr, MD
Fellow, Division of Vascular Surgery, Oregon Health Sciences University,
Portland

Gregory J. Landry, MD
Assistant Professor of Surgery, Division of Vascular Surgery, Oregon
Health Sciences University, Portland

Gregory L. Moneta, MD
Professor of Surgery, Division of Vascular Surgery, Oregon Health
Sciences University, Portland

Lloyd M. Taylor, Jr, MD
Professor of Surgery, Division of Vascular Surgery, Oregon Health
Sciences University, Portland

John M. Porter, MD
Professor of Surgery, Head, Division of Vascular Surgery, Oregon Health
Sciences University, Portland

In their definition of health put forth in 1948, the World Health Organization emphasized not only the absence of disease and infirmity but also the presence of physical, mental, and social well-being. During the last several decades, there has been an increasing focus in medical clinical research on assessing outcomes under this broader definition. In the forefront of this shift in focus was the Medical Outcomes Study, a 2-year observational study conducted in the late 1980s and designed to develop practical tools for monitoring patient outcomes and their determinants.[1]

From this study came some global patient questionnaires designed to assess functional status from the patients' perspective. The Short Form-36 (SF-36) is the best known of these questionnaires and continues to be widely used today (Table 1). Despite its popularity as a global health measure, the SF-36 evaluates deviations from normal health, and is far less sensitive in differentiating varying degrees of chronic illness, a measurement needed to treat the population with peripheral arterial disease, none of whom are healthy. Several other questionnaires also address global health status, including the RAND-36-Item Health Survey 1.0 and the EuroQol.[2-4] The Peripheral Arterial Disease–Walking Impairment Questionnaire is specifically intended for patients with peripheral arterial disease. During the last decade, these questionnaires as well as other methods have been used in assessing vascular surgery outcomes.

BACKGROUND

Traditionally, the results of lower extremity revascularization have been reported using standard parameters of graft patency and limb salvage. Although reports of modern series confirm ever-improving graft patency and limb salvage data, these parameters assess only the technical success of peripheral arterial surgery, which is of obvious importance to the surgeon. Neither parameter permits assessment of the total effect of an operation from the patient's point of view, expressed in terms of functional outcome and quality of life.

Despite the well-documented operative technical success, many physicians have legitimate concerns regarding the appropriate role

TABLE 1.

Assessment Parameters of the Medical
Outcomes Study 36-Item Short-Form[1]

Concept	No. of Items
Physical functioning	10
General health perceptions	5
Mental health	5
Energy/fatigue	4
Role functioning—physical	4
Role functioning—emotional	3
Social functioning	2
Pain	2
Change in health	1

of infrainguinal bypass in limb salvage. Patients with limb-threatening ischemia are frequently nearing the end of life, and most have serious comorbid medical conditions. Because of age and medical conditions, some of these patients already have lost sufficient functional ability to require nursing home placement (8% in a recent study), and it is reasonable to assume that many others are at significant risk for loss of independence. This is one reason why patency and limb salvage are less-than-ideal parameters for assessment of the results of limb salvage surgery, whereas functional outcome and quality of life factors are especially important considerations in this subgroup of vascular patients.

APPROACH IN VASCULAR SURGERY

Recognizing this problem, recent efforts to evaluate the results of lower extremity bypass surgery include assessment of functional outcomes after vascular surgery. The Peripheral Arterial Disease–Walking Impairment Questionnaire developed by Regensteiner et al[2] has been validated for assessment of functional status in patients with claudication. No questionnaire has similarly been validated for assessment of patients with severe limb-threatening ischemia. The RAND-36-Item Health Survey 1.0, which is identical to the Medical Outcomes Study Short Form, was applied to a group of 38 patients undergoing bypass for limb salvage by Duggan et al.[3] These authors found no difference in health perceptions between patients with successful limb salvage and patients with failed bypass grafts requiring amputation, suggesting that this global health assessment instrument is insufficiently sensitive to detect differences in status within a severely diseased population such as that typified by limb salvage patients.

Beyond the fact that no questionnaire has been developed and, more importantly, validated for specifically assessing functional outcome and quality of life issues in patients undergoing limb salvage surgery, questionnaires in general are limited in their power of assessment. They are, by definition, subjective tools of analysis that may be prone to certain biases if not validated for the specific disease process or medical condition being studied. Furthermore, results of questionnaires may be influenced by the timing of their administration in relationship to the event being studied. Lastly, results can vary depending on whether a questionnaire is administered by the physicians or nurses involved in the study patient's care versus independent study personnel.

It is reasonable to assume that the purposes of infrainguinal bypass for limb salvage include elimination of ischemic symp-

TABLE 2.
Objective Parameters for Assessment of Functional Outcome
After Infrainguinal Bypass for Limb Salvage

1. Elimination of ischemic symptoms
2. Operative complications
3. Healing of all wounds—operative and ischemic
4. Recurrence of symptoms
5. Repeat operations
6. Return to preoperative or higher ambulatory level
7. Return to preoperative or higher level of living status

toms, healing of ischemic lesions, preservation of walking ability, and maintenance of patient independent living status. If lower extremity bypass for limb salvage achieves limb preservation at the expense of requiring dependent care or nursing home placement for a significant number of patients previously living independently, it is difficult to justify such a costly surgical intervention. Similarly, for many patients with limb-threatening ischemia, ambulatory function is already seriously impaired. If preservation of ischemic limbs by revascularization is not accompanied by healing of wounds and preservation of ambulation, successful limb salvage has little functional meaning. A final consideration is the need for and frequency of repeat interventions to treat new or recurrent symptoms. Quality of life is negatively impacted if limb salvage surgery is followed by multiple interventions so that a significant portion of the patient's remaining lifetime is spent in hospitals, clinics, or "temporary" care facilities. These factors—resolution of symptoms, wound healing, ambulatory status, living status, and the need for repeat intervention—are the minimum objective data required to assess functional outcome and quality-of-life issues in patients undergoing limb salvage surgery (Table 2).

CURRENT DATA

Our approach to assessing quality of life and functional outcomes in patients undergoing limb salvage surgery has, therefore, focused not on patient questionnaires but on the objective factors described above. Initially, we performed a study of outcomes in patients after revascularization of threatened limbs in which functional outcome was defined in terms of a minimally acceptable therapeutic result.[5] The functional outcome was evaluated in terms of independence in living status and ambulatory ability. These are factors which, if not preserved, define an undesirable outcome of the surgery, independent of graft patency and preservation of the limb. Evaluation of functional status preoperatively and 6 months post-operatively was performed in 613 patients who underwent infrain-guinal bypass for limb salvage (Table 3). This period was chosen to allow for healing of ischemic wounds and for temporary nursing home placement, which is frequently required by third-party pay-ers as a lower-cost alternative to prolonged hospitalization. At the same time, 6 months was sufficiently soon after the index opera-tion that deterioration of functional status and quality of life from comorbid conditions was minimized.

Infrainguinal bypass for limb salvage achieved the goal of main-taining independent living and ambulation in the vast majority of those treated who survived 6 months. Ninety-six percent of sur-vivors who were both living independently and ambulatory pre-operatively continued to be so 6 months postoperatively. Not surprisingly, preoperative living status and ability to ambulate were the most important factors predictive of postoperative func-tional status. Unfortunately, the status of patients who were living in nursing homes or nonambulatory preoperatively was rarely improved by limb salvage surgery. Only one patient recovered to independent living status postoperatively from a preoperative nursing home status, and only 6 of 29 patients (21%) who were nonambulatory preoperatively became ambulatory postoperatively (Fig 1). Although there may be compelling reasons to consider limb revascularization in nursing home or nonambulatory patients,

TABLE 3.

Functional Status of Surviving Patients Before Surgery and 6 Months After Infrainguinal Bypass for Limb Salvage

Before Surgery	6 Months After Surgery	
Living situation	Independent	Dependent
Independent	99%	1.4%
Dependent	4%	96%
Ambulatory status	Ambulatory	Nonambulatory
Ambulatory	97%	3%
Nonambulatory	21%	79%
Living independently and ambulatory	Living independently and ambulatory 96%	

(Courtesy of Abou-Zamzam AM Jr, Lee RW, Moneta GL, et al: Functional outcome after infrainguinal bypass for limb salvage. *J Vasc Surg* 25:287-297, 1997. Reprinted with per-mission.)

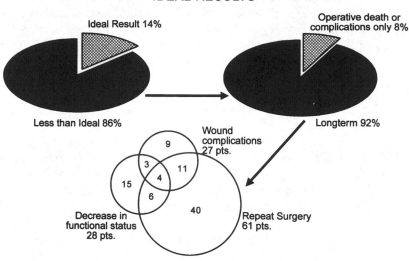

INFRAINGUINAL BYPASS FOR LIMB SALVAGE
IDEAL RESULTS

FIGURE 1.
Only 16 of 112 patients (14%) achieved an ideal result. Of the 96 patients who failed to achieve an ideal result, 8 (8%) failed because of perioperative death or complications only, and 88 (92%) failed because of long-term factors. Sixty-one of the 96 patients (64%) required repeat surgery, 28 (29%) had a decrease in functional status (ambulatory or living status), and 27 (28%) had wound complications. (Courtesy of Nicoloff AD, Taylor LM Jr, McLafferty RB, et al: Patient recovery after infrainguinal bypass grafting for limb salvage. *J Vasc Surg* 27:256-266, 1998. Reprinted with permission.)

these results suggest that such procedures should be considered carefully, because return to independent living, ambulation, or both is usually not achievable.

Although functional outcome at 6 months appeared encouraging, patients who had undergone infrainguinal bypass for limb salvage on our service appeared to follow a clinical course characterized by a frequent and ongoing need for care, including repeat hospitalizations for wound care and repeat surgery. Even those not requiring subsequent operations or hospitalizations often were still suffering because of prolonged healing of their ischemic and operative wounds. In other words, it appeared that a significant portion of the remaining lives of patients undergoing revascularization for limb salvage was spent dealing with ongoing care of their limbs. An attempt to characterize and quantify these clinical observations, familiar to many surgeons, constituted the basis for further study.

From a patient's perspective, the ideal outcome after infrainguinal bypass surgery is to undergo a single successful operation with no complications, have prompt resolution of symptoms and wound healing, and require no further operations or interventions for peripheral ischemia. It is our belief that to the patient it matters little whether a repeat operation required after initially successful infrainguinal bypass for limb salvage is performed on the contralateral limb for new symptoms, or on the ipsilateral limb for a wound problem, for revision of a graft stenosis, or for recurrent ischemia caused by development of a stenosis in the inflow vessel, although each of these events affects traditional parameters that assess the results of the original operation quite differently. As the patient sees it, repeat hospitalization and surgery, postoperative wound healing, and the necessary clinic visits are indistinguishable from the original episode of ischemia. In other words, patients view the entire ordeal, operation and recovery, as "the problem" and their functional outcome should be assessed accordingly.

The records of 112 consecutive patients who underwent initial infrainguinal bypass for limb salvage 5 to 7 years before the time of the study were reviewed for operative complications, graft patency, limb salvage, survival, patient functional status (living situation, ambulatory status), time to achieve wound healing (both operative and ischemic), need for repeat operations, and recurrence of ischemia.[6] Mean postoperative follow-up was 42 months. Preoperatively, 99 patients (88%) lived independently at home and 103 (92%) were ambulatory. There were 7 (6%) perioperative deaths, and wound complications occurred in 27 patients (24%). By life-table, assisted primary graft patency and limb salvage of the index extremity 5 years postoperatively were 77% and 87% respectively, whereas patient survival was 49% at 5 years (Table 4). At last follow-up or death, 73% of the patients (72/99) who lived independently at home preoperatively were still living independently at home, whereas 70% (72/103) of those who were ambulatory preoperatively remained ambulatory. Before surgery, 86% (96/112) were ambulatory and living independently at home. Of these 96 patients, 68% were ambulatory and living independently at home at the time of last follow-up or death (Table 5).

Healing of all wounds, both operative and ischemic, required a mean of 4.2 months (Table 6). Twenty-five patients (22%) had not achieved complete wound healing at the time of last follow-up or death. Repeat operations to maintain graft patency, treat wound

TABLE 4.

Life Table Analysis of Conventional Measures of 112 Patients After Limb Salvage Surgery

	Assisted Primary Patency (SE)	Limb Salvage (SE)	Survival (SE)
6 months	93.1% (0.03)	94.9% (0.02)	81.3% (0.04)
3 years	87.6% (0.04)	93.5% (0.03)	61.8% (0.05)
5 years	77.3% (0.05)	86.9% (0.04)	49.0% (0.05)

(Courtesy of Nicoloff AD, Taylor LM Jr, McLafferty RB, et al: Patient recovery after infrainguinal bypass grafting for limb salvage. *J Vasc Surg* 27:256-266, 1998. Reprinted with permission.)

complications, or treat recurrent or contralateral ischemia were required in 61 patients (54%) (mean, 1.6 reoperations per patient) (Table 7). This did not include the initial debridement or minor amputation if required and performed as a separate operation. Twenty-six patients (23.2%) ultimately required major limb amputation of the index or contralateral extremity. Only 16 of 112 patients (14.3%) achieved the ideal surgical result of an uncomplicated operation with elimination of symptoms, maintenance of functional status, and no recurrence of ischemia or need for repeat operations (Fig 1).

It was not the purpose of this recent study to suggest that the rapidly declining functional status and poor long-term survival documented in the limb salvage patient group were entirely or even primarily caused by either lower extremity ischemia or by the surgery performed for its treatment. Clearly, this was not the case. Rather, limb-threatening ischemia is a manifestation of ath-

TABLE 5.

Ambulatory and Living Status of 112 Patients Before and After Limb Salvage Surgery

	Preoperative Status	Postoperative Status	Status at Last Follow-up or Death
Living independently	88% (99/112)	66% (66/99)	73% (72/99)
Ambulatory	92% (103/112)	84% (87/103)	70% (72/103)
Living independently and ambulatory	86% (96/112)	56% (54/96)	68% (65/96)

TABLE 6.

Wound Healing Time (in Months) of Operative and Ischemic Wounds*

	Operative Wounds	Ischemic Wounds	All Wounds
Mean	1.9	5.2	4.2
Median	1.3	3.4	2.7
Range	0.4-10.1	0.4-48.3	0.4-48.3

*Data only include wounds that healed completely.

erosclerosis that occurs in patients approaching the end of life, at a time when functional status is frequently declining rapidly and interval survival is short. This study makes clear that this state of affairs is improved very little by surgical intervention for the treatment of limb-threatening ischemia.

Our 1997 study summarized above, as well as those from other institutions, suggests that patient ambulatory status and living situation (parameters most directly related to limb salvage) are maintained shortly after bypass surgery.[5,7] That this is not the case for a considerable number of patients in the long-term is clearly documented in our 1998 study, in which only 68% of patients who were ambulatory and living independently before surgery maintained this status at the time of last follow-up or death.

TABLE 7.

Repeat Operations*

Type of Operation	Total No. (%)
Wound debridement	32 (18.2)
Minor amputation	26 (14.8)
Skin grafting	3 (1.7)
Major amputation	26 (14.8)
New graft construction	42 (23.8)
Graft revisions	32 (18.2)
Inflow procedures	15 (8.5)
Total	176 (100)

*Figures include repeat operations to maintain graft patency; to treat ongoing, recurrent, or contralateral ischemia; or to treat wound complications. Figures do not include 40 subsequent operations performed to treat the original ischemic lesions.
(Courtesy of Nicoloff AD, Taylor LM Jr, McLafferty RB, et al: Patient recovery after infrainguinal bypass grafting for limb salvage. *J Vasc Surg* 27:256-266, 1998. Reprinted with permission.)

As assessed by the objective of the "ideal outcome," optimal results of infrainguinal bypass for limb salvage are distinctly infrequent. Only 14% of patients had an uncomplicated operation, relief of symptoms, complete wound healing, no need for repeat surgery, and maintenance of functional status. For the 86% of patients who did not have ideal results, wound care, repeat hospitalizations and repeat surgery, frequent clinic visits, and declining functional status meant that a major feature of their remaining life was ongoing treatment for limb ischemia.

CONCLUSION

We conclude that although clinically important palliation is frequently achieved by infrainguinal bypass for limb salvage, ideal results are distinctly infrequent. Methods of assessing outcomes continue to be developed and, to be complete, will need to use a combination of surveys, functional assessments, and surgical results. Most patients undergoing infrainguinal bypass for limb salvage require continued or repeated treatment for a significant portion of their remaining lives. In view of these results, we must be certain patients and their referring physicians are aware of the ongoing and palliative nature of the care that will be required to treat their limb ischemia. Continued evaluation of alternative approaches to therapy, including nonoperative treatment and primary amputation, appears warranted. While we have successfully spent the past several decades defining the technical limits of what can be done surgically to treat limb-threatening ischemia, we are now entering a new era of defining when such surgery should be done.

REFERENCES

1. Ware JE Jr, Sherbourne CD: The MOS 36-item short-form health survey (SF-36): I. Conceptual framework and item selection. *Med Care* 30:473-483, 1992.
2. Regensteiner JG, Steiner JF, Panzer RJ, et al: Evaluation of walking impairment by questionnaire in patients with peripheral arterial disease. *J Vasc Med Biol* 2:142-152, 1990.
3. Duggan MM, Woodsen J, Scott TE, et al: Functional outcome in limb salvage vascular surgery. *Am J Surg* 168:188-191, 1994.
4. The EuroQol Group: A new facility for the measurement of health-related quality of life. *Health Policy* 16:199-208, 1990.
5. Abou-Zamzam AM Jr, Lee RW, Moneta GL, et al: Functional outcome after infrainguinal bypass for limb salvage. *J Vasc Surg* 25:287-297, 1997.
6. Nicoloff AD, Taylor LM Jr, McLafferty RB, et al: Patient recovery after

infrainguinal bypass grafting for limb salvage. *J Vasc Surg* 27:256-266, 1998.

7. Pomposelli FB Jr, Arora S, Gibbons GW, et al: Lower extremity arterial reconstruction in the very elderly: Successful outcome preserves not only the limb but also residential status and ambulatory function. *J Vasc Surg* 28:215-225, 1998.

PART IV

Access for Hemodialysis

CHAPTER 8

Management of Iatrogenic Complications From Arterial Access

Giuseppe R. Nigri, MD
Research Fellow in Vascular Surgery, Massachusetts General Hospital,
Harvard Medical School, Boston

Glenn M. LaMuraglia, MD
Associate Professor of Surgery, Massachusetts General Hospital, Harvard
Medical School, Boston

Complications after diagnostic and therapeutic catheterization procedures are becoming more common as the number of complex invasive procedures performed increases.[1] Peripheral arteriography with the use of direct puncture was introduced in 1929. In 1953 Seldinger introduced a percutaneous technique with the use of a guidewire for introduction and exchange of catheters in the arterial system. This method revolutionized percutaneous access, and today it forms the basis of most arterial access procedures (blood pressure monitoring and peripheral and cardiac diagnostic and interventional procedures).

Unlike a diagnostic intra-arterial study, larger catheters are required for complex interventional procedures such as percutaneous transluminal angioplasty, stenting, valvuloplasty, or intra-aortic balloon pump placement. These interventions may also require anticoagulation, intravascular manipulations, and the occasional deployment of devices. These "less invasive" procedures are not without complications, and can be associated with bleeding, thromboembolism, dissection, AV fistula, and infection.

ROUTE OF ARTERIAL ACCESS
TRANSFEMORAL ACCESS

The most common site for arterial access is the femoral artery. It is a relatively large vessel, superficial in svelte persons, easy to cannulate, not adjacent to vulnerable structures, and its location over the femoral head allows easy compression of the femoral artery to provide hemostasis after catheter removal. There is also a sheath around the common femoral that provides additional structural support to limit bleeding after catheter removal.

Although catheters up to 14F ($F = d \times \pi$) or 4.4 mm in diameter have been successfully used to percutaneously access the femoral artery, the complications are correlated to the size of the introduced device. The incidence of complications after percutaneous diagnostic procedures is about 0.7%, whereas the incidence of those related to percutaneous interventional procedures, which require a larger sheath, is approximately 3%.[2]

The presence of a prosthetic bypass graft usually does not contraindicate femoral access for cannulation. Use of the groin in patients who have undergone an aortofemoral bypass graft or femoral-popliteal grafts can be safe when judiciously approached and when no anastomotic aneurysms are present. Even an intra-aortic balloon pump can be safely placed percutaneously using a large sheath into aorto-femoral grafts.[3] However, using arterial access with the femoral approach in the presence of a femoral to femoral graft is fraught with possible complications. The angle and position of this graft predispose to anastomotic injury during puncture and, should the injury result in thrombosis, ischemia can develop in both lower extremities.

UPPER EXTREMITY ACCESS

When femoral access is unavailable because of occlusive disease or other circumstances, secondary arterial access sites can be selected in the upper extremities. However, upper extremity arterial access involves catheters crossing the aortic arch, which raises the infrequent complication of stroke.

Recently, access through the radial artery has been popularized for cardiac catheterization access in patients with a normal Allen test result. No major veins or nerves surround the artery, minimizing the chance of injury to adjacent structures. The radial artery is superficial, and hemostasis can be achieved by simple compression of the artery on the radius or using specifically designed occlusive tourniquets at the puncture site. This approach is optimally performed with long sheaths up to 7F in size, which facilitate catheter exchanges at the level of the brachial artery. Transradial catheterization has been reported to significantly reduce the median length of hospital stay by allowing early patient mobilization. However, the possibility of radial artery injury and occlusion (5%) still remains appreciable, reducing its use as a possible coronary artery bypass conduit or arterial line monitoring site.[4]

The approach through the "axillary artery" is generally through the proximal brachial artery in the arm. The percutaneous brachial access can be difficult to perform because of the small size and mobility of this vessel and often results in patient discomfort. Frequently, a surgical cutdown, referred to as the Sones technique, is undertaken. Thrombosis, related to the relatively small diameter of the brachial artery, is a frequent complication but it is well tolerated because of the large collateral network in the arm. True axillary artery access is rarely used because of difficulty with compression after catheter removal, and bleeding can easily result in brachial plexus nerve compression and injury.

COMPLICATIONS AND THEIR MANAGEMENT

Complications of percutaneous intra-arterial access can be classified as systemic or site related (Table 1). During percutaneous arterial procedures, a vasovagal reaction is the most common systemic complication and consists of hypotension, bradycardia, nausea, pallor, and diaphoresis—all signs that can be readily misinterpreted as bleeding. During coronary access, these findings can mimic cardiac problems, and the patient should be carefully evaluated to determine the cause, if any, of these findings. The vasovagal response is generally self-limited and often resolves with fluid administration; atropine is rarely necessary.

Spontaneous bleeding at locations remote from the puncture site can occur during arterial access procedures because of thrombolysis and anticoagulation. Bleeding can occur in the retroperitoneum on the same or opposite side to the femoral puncture, in skeletal muscles (eg, rectus muscle), or intracranially. Patients should be observed or treated depending on their clinical manifestations, while stopping the anticoagulation.

The complications related to the catheter site include bleeding, thrombosis, embolization, AV fistula, nerve injury and infection.

BLEEDING

Bleeding is the most common complication after any arterial access. It is correlated to the size of the sheath and the ratio between the size of the hole and the caliber of the artery. Therefore, bleeding is more common in females than males because of the smaller size of their arteries. This causative factor is less prevalent with technological advances that have reduced the

TABLE 1.

Complications From Arterial Access

1. Complications not related to catheter site
    Vasovagal syndrome
    Spontaneous bleeding (retroperitoneal, rectus muscle, intracranial)
    Renal failure
    Cardiac (myocardial infarction, congestive heart failure)
2. Complications related to catheter site
Bleeding
Risk factors
    Ratio hole size/artery caliber
    Smaller body surface area, shorter height, lighter weight
    Sex (more common in females who have smaller arteries)
    Size of sheath (larger in complex invasive technique)
    Position of the hole (anterior vs side)
    Catheterization of a side branch
    Site of puncture (low or high site of puncture related to inguinal ligament)
    PFA angle
    Peripheral vascular disease
Poor hemostasis
    Poor technique
    Abundant subcutaneous tissue
    Difficult compression (hematoma, patient motion)
    Aortic insufficiency (friable vessel)
Coagulation factors
    Antiplatelet and anticoagulation therapy (heparin, coumadin, integrin
      inhibitor)
    Coagulopathy
    Inadequate monitoring after the procedure
Hypertension
    Inadequate BP control and monitoring
Complications of bleeding
    Pseudoaneurysm
    Retroperitoneal bleeding
    Shock
Thrombosis
    Excessive compression at the access site
    Artery dissection, plaque disruption
    Inadequate anticoagulation: thrombus on sheath, catheter, IABP, mal-
      functions of hemostatic device
    Bypass graft
    Small arterial size (brachial and radial access)
Embolization
Plaque disruption
    — Femoral and iliac artery

(continued)

TABLE 1. (continued)

—   Abdominal aortic aneurysm
—   Aortic arch

AV fistula
Usually asymptomatic
Holosystolic/diastolic bruit

Nerve injury
Direct nerve injury
—   Puncture during anesthetic injection
—   Puncture during catheterization
Pseudoaneurysm or hematoma nerve compression
Retroperitoneal bleeding
Scar involving the nerve

Infection
Gross contamination of material
Prolonged indwelling sheaths (eg, stroke thrombolysis)

Abbreviations: PFA, profunda femoral artery; *BP*, blood pressure; *IABP*, intraaortic balloon pump; *AV*, arteriovenous.

sheath sizes; today, a coronary artery stenting can be performed with a 6F introducer sheath, and an intraaortic balloon pump can be placed with a 9.5F introducer.

Other risk factors for bleeding during arterial access include cannulating through a side branch of the artery or through the side of the artery wall. Both occurrences prevent adequate compression for sealing of the artery access site. Location of the arterial puncture is also important. If the puncture site is above the inguinal ligament, effective compression cannot be achieved because of its deep location in the pelvis and the damping effect when pressure is applied on the inguinal ligament or the abdominal wall. A puncture distal to the femoral artery can cause bleeding from another mechanism. If the profunda femoral artery is cannulated, the relatively rigid sheath can tear the artery during insertion because of its upward angle, enlarging the size of the arterial puncture site and resulting in bleeding during the procedure (Fig 1). The smaller size of the superficial and profunda femoral artery in comparison with the common femoral artery results in a large puncture hole to vessel diameter ratio, increasing the likelihood of bleeding. The presence of a hematoma or abundant subcutaneous tissue decreases the ability to effectively compress the artery after sheath removal, resulting in a higher likelihood of increased blood loss (Fig 2).

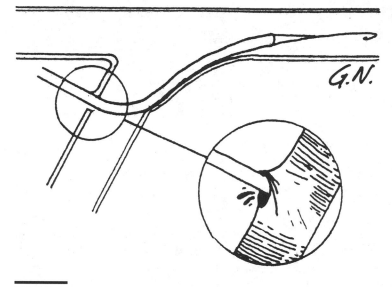

FIGURE 1.
By cannulating the profunda femoral artery, the relatively rigid sheath can tear the artery during insertion because of its upward angle, enlarging the size of the arterial puncture site and resulting in bleeding during the procedure.

Bleeding also correlates with the inhibition of the clotting cascade. Antiplatelet and anticoagulant treatment (heparin, coumadin, integrin inhibitors) or coagulopathies increase the incidence of blood loss. The presence of elevated blood pressure or of aortic insufficiency, with a high difference in pressure per period of time and more friable vessels, also contributes to the likelihood of bleeding. Meticulous technique and patient cooperation are also important factors in achieving good hemostasis after sheath removal.

To prevent these bleeding complications in anticoagulated patients, hemostatic devices have been developed for use at the time of sheath removal. These include hemostatic collagen plugs, which close the puncture site by promoting platelet adhesion and clot formation. The early collagen plugs could easily dislodge from the deployed location, resulting in delayed bleeding, arterial occlusion, or distal embolization.[5] The new collagen plugs (Angio-Seal) (Fig 3) can be secured into the desired position by the means of an intravascular absorbable anchor.[6] This diminishes the likelihood of embolization or thrombosis and improves hemostasis. However, all the collagen plugs prevent access through the same vessel for a certain time after placement. Another device (Fig 4) developed for diminishing bleeding after sheath removal is the suture-mediated vascular closure system (Perclose). This device allows percutaneous closure of the artery at the puncture site by a surgical suturing technique. Although these devices decrease postinterventional bed rest and hospital stay, and diminish bleeding complications, they are not without their own complications, which can usually result in failure to stop bleeding or result in arterial obstruction (Fig 5).

Among the bleeding complications, hematoma accounts for approximately 6% and pseudoaneurysms (PSAs) for 0.5% to 9% of cases.[7] The most common bleeding complication of femoral access that requires treatment is the PSA. It is a pulsatile hematoma that communicates with the circulation through the puncture in the arterial wall which has not sealed. PSAs are associated with a local early systolic bruit, but depending on the patient's body habitus or the presence of a hematoma, palpation of the lesion may be difficult. The definitive diagnosis can be made by ultrasonography.

The PSA is connected to the artery by a neck whose diameter and length can vary considerably (Fig 6, *A*). Short broad necks

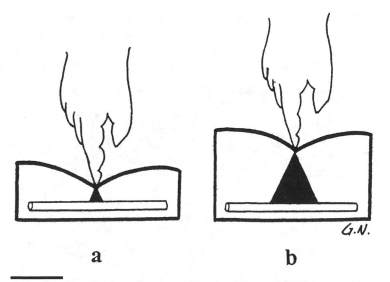

a   b

FIGURE 2.

A, In svelte patients, compression is often effective because the pressure is localized to a small area *(shaded area).* **B,** The presence of a hematoma or abundant subcutaneous fat decreases the ability to effectively compress the artery after sheath removal and provides a larger distribution of pressure *(shaded area).*

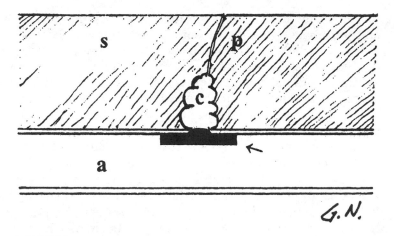

FIGURE 3.
New-generation collagen plug hemostatic device. *Arrow,* absorbable anchor; *c,* collagen plug; *p,* puncture tract; *s,* subcutaneous tissue; *a,* artery.

make compression therapy difficult (Fig 6, *B*), whereas thin necks make compression effective to thrombose the PSA (Fig 6, *C*). Although spontaneous occlusion of untreated PSAs (89%) has been reported,[8] this can take time to occur, and rupture and bleeding of the PSA can cause significant morbidity and (rarely) death.

In the past, the treatment of femoral PSA has traditionally been surgical. However, today most PSAs can be successfully treated

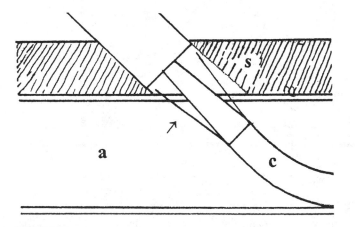

FIGURE 4.
Suture-mediated vascular closure device. The needles (arrow) are engaged in the vessel wall in order to close the arterial puncture site. *S,* subcutaneous tissue; *a,* artery; *c,* catheter.

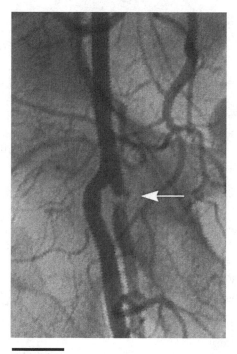

FIGURE 5.
Angiogram of a patient with an obstructed superficial femoral artery *(arrow)* resulting from a suture-mediated vascular closure device.

with external compression to induce thrombosis. In our experience, if a PSA is identified after a catheterization by the presence of a new bruit or a pulsatile mass at the site of the puncture, the next step is the directed external compression of the PSA. If the diagnosis is unclear, the presence of a PSA requires confirmation by ultrasound.

Directed external PSA compression is done on the unfed patient (to avoid possible aspiration) who is sedated and given local anesthesia. The anesthetic (1% xylocaine) is injected into the overlaying skin with care to avoid intravascular injection. A C-clamp is applied for 30 to 40 minutes over the presumed location of the arterial puncture. The area of compression is the point at which the arterial puncture is judged to have taken place (based on skin puncture and pulsatile mass location) and not necessarily at the apex of the PSA. However, other devices such as a Femostop can be used.[9] During the procedure, perfusion of the lower extremity is carefully monitored. The clamp must be slowly released over minutes to avoid acutely filling the PSA tract. The patient is evaluated by physical examination or by ultrasound depending on the findings. For initial failures, the procedure can be repeated several times to induce thrombosis. Patients should be kept at bed rest for 4 to 6 hours after the compression and slowly mobilized. This procedure has been successful in most non-anticoagulated patients. The presence of a bypass graft, signs of skin ischemia, or signs of local infection contraindicate the use of compression. Although ultrasound-guided compression has been successfully reported,[10,11] in our experience it has not been necessary to commit the resources of a technician and an ultrasound machine to achieve successful thrombosis of the PSA, but it is generally used when directed external compression has failed.

Ultrasound-guided thrombin injection has been recently reported.[1,12] Although fast and effective, this should be limited to patients with PSA resulting from diagnostic studies without critical anatomy or recent intervention such as angioplasty or stent. Thrombin is a potent activator of platelets that can theoretically result in platelet deposition at the interventional site, resulting in thrombosis. Although this technique has been advocated for all PSAs, we routinely use it only when a patient has had a diagnostic study without critical anatomy.

Recently, PSAs have been treated by percutaneous implantation of endovascular polyester fabric–covered nitinol stents.[7] Although this is an intriguing concept, the placement of a stent in the femoral artery at the level of a joint appears to be injudicious, with potential complications and the rendering of that artery inaccessible to

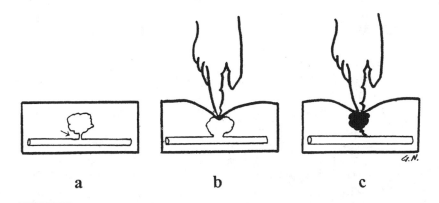

a   b   c

FIGURE 6.
The pseudoaneurysm (PSA) is connected to the artery by a neck **(A)**. Short, broad necks make compression therapy difficult **(B)**, whereas thin necks make compression effective to thrombose the PSA **(C)**.

Reservation Card for Advances

Yes! I would like my own copy of *Advances in Vascular Surgery®, Volume 8* (ISSN 1069-7292) at the price of **$88.00** (**$94.00** outside the U.S.) plus sales tax, postage, and handling. Please begin my subscription with the current edition according to the terms described below.* I understand that I will have 30 days to examine each annual edition.

Name _____

Address _____

City _____ State_____ ZIP _____

Method of Payment

❑ Check (in U.S. dollars, drawn on a U.S. bank, payable to **Mosby**)

❑ VISA   ❑ MasterCard   ❑ AmEx   ❑ Bill me

Card number _____ Exp. date _____

Signature _____

Prices are subject to change without notice.

MO144/D51599

Subscribe to the related journal in your field!

Full-text Online Access Included!

Yes! Begin my one-year subscription to *Journal of Vascular Surgery* (Volumes 31-32, 2000, 12 issues, ISSN 0741-5214). Full-text online access is included for all print subscribers.

Name _____

Institution _____

Address _____

City _____ State_____

ZIP/PC _____ Country _____

E-mail _____

Subscription prices

	USA	Int'l
Individuals ❑	$177.00	$215.00
Institutions ❑	330.00	368.00
Students/residents† ❑	91.00	129.00

Method of payment

❑ Check (in U.S. dollars, drawn on a U.S. bank, and payable to *Mosby*).

❑ VISA   ❑ MasterCard

❑ AmEx   ❑ Bill me   Exp. date_____

Card # _____

Signature _____

†Please supply, on institution letterhead, your name, dates of study/residency, and signature of program coordinator. Orders will be billed at the individual rate until proof of status is received.

Airmail rates available upon request.
Prices subject to change without notice.

MO144/D51607

---

*Your Advances service guarantee:

When you subscribe to *Advances*, you will receive advance notice of future annual volumes about two months before publication. To receive the new edition, you need do nothing—we'll send you the new volume as soon as it is available. If you want to discontinue, the advance notice allows you time to notify us of your decision. If you are not completely satisfied, you have 30 days to return any *Advances*.

further catheterization procedures. This is especially true because other safe therapies are readily available.

Surgical repair is straightforward and can be undertaken with safety even in ill patients. The skin is initially cleansed with hydrogen peroxide, to remove coagulated blood and protein to minimize wound infections, and then prepared in standard fashion. Local anesthetic is administered under sedation. The incision is carried through the PSA, and digital control of bleeding is obtained directly over the artery puncture site without previously obtaining proximal or distal arterial control. The artery wall is subsequently well exposed by dissecting above and below the puncture site. Judd-Allis clamps are placed directly on the artery wall in a transverse fashion to align the arteriotomy edges atraumatically. Simple interrupted 5-0 polypropylene sutures are used to close the artery while removing the Judd-Allis clamps. The use of a prosthetic patch is discouraged and avoided because it can be a source of infection and the suture line can be disrupted at future catheterization procedures, resulting in bleeding. Lastly, the posterior wall of the artery is exposed to ensure there is no posterior bleeding site. The hematoma is evacuated and the wound is closed primarily. No drains are used because they generally promote a lymph leak for extended periods and may contribute to late infections. Large cavities can be compressed by a 6-inch Ace wrap applied from the foot to the groin crease and left on for several days. The patients are generally mobilized after 24 hours unless they had a very large cavity or hematoma. This approach is used for simple PSAs but should not be used when infection is suspected or a late bleeding complication occurs. The presence of a prior primary surgical PSA artery repair is not a contraindication of arterial access for interventional procedures.

An insidious and potentially dangerous complication is retroperitoneal bleeding with little evidence of local swelling or hematoma. This is particularly common in patients with prior groin surgery that precludes the development of a larger hematoma because of scar tissue. Patients with retroperitoneal bleeding may complain of abdominal and back pain or femoral neuralgia and leg pain, but usually they are relatively asymptomatic until hypotension appears or the hematocrit decreases. Diagnosis is confirmed by pelvic computed tomography scan. Generally, the retroperitoneal bleeding resolves spontaneously after supportive therapy. Surgical exploration for decompression of hematoma is indicated in the presence of PSA and retroperitoneal bleeding, and it is mandatory when there is nerve root entrapment.

THROMBOSIS AND EMBOLIZATION

The possibility of thrombosis is inversely related to the diameter of the vessel and directly related to the diameter of the sheath. This condition is less common with femoral access than with upper extremity access. Furthermore, the incidence of thrombosis is decreased with the introduction of smaller and smaller sheaths and the widespread use of anticoagulation therapy. Another condition that can lead to thrombosis includes the overcompression of an artery and especially overcompression of a prosthetic graft after sheath removal.

Arterial dissection can also cause thrombosis and vessel obstruction. Iatrogenic dissection occurs more commonly in the iliac vessels because of their tortuosity and the high incidence of atherosclerotic occlusive disease. Prevention of arterial dissection consists of using appropriate catheters and wires that must be advanced through the lumen under continuous fluoroscopic control. Usually a retrograde dissection resolves after catheter removal because the flap is raised opposite to the direction of blood flow. Occasionally, deployment of a stent may be necessary to treat a progressive or symptomatic arterial dissection in the iliac arteries.

Embolic events are more commonly related to plaque disruption caused by catheter abrading of atherosclerotic intimal surfaces. Depending on their location, patients can have "blue toe" syndrome, decreased perfusion of the extremities, or renal failure. Although large emboli are treated with surgical embolectomy, micro-emboli can only be treated by ensuring optimal circulation to the affected extremity for ultimate heeling of the lesion.

AV FISTULA

An AV fistula is a consequence of an injury involving both the artery and the adjacent vein. Usually the superficial femoral artery or the profunda femoral artery is involved. AV fistulas are generally asymptomatic, and their discovery is usually incidental.

The pathognomonic sign of an AV fistula is a holosystolic/diastolic bruit over the catheter site. No other diagnostic tests are needed. AV fistulas generally close spontaneously and should be followed up to ensure they do not grow to become a clinical problem. Therefore, if the ejection fraction is in good range and the patient has no cardiac heart failure, no therapy other than follow-up is needed. Surgical treatment includes the repair of both the artery and the vein with the placement of soft tissue between the suture lines.

NERVE INJURY

Rarely, the femoral nerve can be injured accessing the femoral artery. When injury to the femoral nerve occurs, it usually results from the anesthesia injection directly into the nerve. It can also be related to direct puncture during cannulation. Indirect nerve injury results from compression caused by a hematoma or a PSA impinging on the nerve. This can occur in the groin or in the retroperitoneum, depending on the anatomical location of the bleeding. Patients with nerve injury generally have pain and may have motor weakness and sensory loss, with absence of a knee jerk and diminished sensation over the anterior and medial thigh. To examine the motor component of the femoral nerve, the posterior knee is supported while the patient straightens the leg. The ability to bend the knee by applying downward pressure on the ankle signifies injury or pressure of the femoral nerve. Nerve injury can also occur during upper extremity arterial access and usually affects the median nerve. The treatment of nerve compression is considered a surgical emergency, the aim of which is to evacuate the hematoma causing the pressure-injury and to control the bleeding.

INFECTION

Infection is a rare complication of arterial access. It generally results from a break in sterile technique. Prolonged use of indwelling sheaths such as during intracranial thrombolysis for stroke or intraaortic balloon pump placement in patients undergoing cardiac transplantation can lead to the development of an infection. The infection can involve the soft tissues; in this case, intravenous antibiotics and draining of a fluid collection, if present, is indicated. If the artery has been involved and disrupted by the infectious process, artery replacement and coverage with muscle flaps (sartorius in the groin) is indicated while antibiotics are administered. Resection and extraanatomical bypass (such as obturator bypass in groin) is sometimes indicated in severe purulent infections.

CONCLUSIONS

With the number of diagnostic and interventional procedures requiring percutaneous arterial access increasing, the complications related to arterial access must not be underestimated. The use of the smallest sheath possible for the procedure and minimizing excessive manipulations are strongly recommended to avoid problems. Meticulous technique during the procedure and careful patient observation afterwards will decrease complications of this ever-increasing modality of vascular diagnosis and therapy.

REFERENCES

1. Brophy DP, Sheiman RG, Amatulle P, et al: Iatrogenic femoral pseudoaneurysms: Thrombin injection after failed US-guided compression. *Radiology* 214:278-282, 2000.
2. Messina LM, Brothers TE, Wakefield TW, et al: Clinical characteristics and surgical management of vascular complications in patients undergoing cardiac catheterization: Interventional versus diagnostic procedures. *J Vasc Surg* 13:593-600, 1991.
3. LaMuraglia GM, Vlahakes GJ, Moncure AC, et al: The safety of intraaortic balloon pump catheter insertion through suprainguinal prosthetic vascular bypass grafts. *J Vasc Surg* 13:830-837, 1991.
4. Kiemeneij F, Laarman GJ, Odekerken D, et al: A randomized comparison of percutaneous transluminal coronary angioplasty by the radial, brachial and femoral approaches: The access study. *J Am Coll Cardiol* 29:1269-1275, 1997.
5. Duda SH, Wiskirchen J, Erb M, et al: Suture-mediated percutaneous closure of antegrade femoral arterial access sites in patients who have received full anticoagulation therapy. *Radiology* 210:47-52, 1999.
6. Kussmaul WG, Buchbinder M, Whitlow PL, et al: Femoral artery hemostasis using an implantable device (Angio-Seal) after coronary angioplasty. *Cathet Cardiovasc Diagn* 37:362-365, 1996.
7. Thalhammer C, Kirchherr AS, Uhlich F, et al: Postcatheterization pseudoaneurysms and arteriovenous fistulas: Repair with percutaneous implantation of endovascular covered stents. *Radiology*, 214:127-131, 2000.
8. Toursarkissian B, Allen BT, Petrinec D, et al: Spontaneous closure of selected iatrogenic pseudoaneurysms and arteriovenous fistulae. *J Vasc Surg* 25:803-808, 1997.
9. Chatterjee T, Do DD, Mahler F, et al: Prospective, randomized evaluation of nonsurgical closure of femoral pseudoaneurysm by compression device with or without ultrasound guidance. *Cathet Cardiovasc Intervent* 47:304A-309A, 1999.
10. Dean SM, Olin JW, Piedmonte M, et al: Ultrasound-guided compression closure of postcatheterization pseudoaneurysms during concurrent anticoagulation: A review of seventy-seven patients. *J Vasc Surg* 23:28-34, 1996.
11. Fellmeth BD, Roberts AC, Bookstein JJ, et al: Postangiographic femoral artery injuries: Nonsurgical repair with US-guided compression. *Radiology* 178:671-675, 1991.
12. Kang SS, Labropoulos N, Mansour MA, et al: Expanded indications for ultrasound-guided thrombin injection of pseudoaneurysms. *J Vasc Surg* 31:289-298, 2000.

CHAPTER 9

Basilic Vein Transposition for Chronic Hemodialysis

Albert G. Hakaim, MD
Associate Professor of Surgery, Mayo Medical School, Director,
Endovascular Surgery, St. Luke's Hospital, Jacksonville, Florida

W. Andrew Oldenburg, MD
Assistant Professor of Surgery, Mayo Medical School, Head, Section of
Vascular Surgery, St. Luke's Hospital, Jacksonville, Florida

The two principles guiding creation of arteriovenous access for chronic hemodialysis have remained intact for many years. First, the most durable access should be selected for the initial procedure to provide the longest interval of intervention-free patency. A recent study proved that patients initiated on dialysis with inadequate access function, from either an autogenous arteriovenous fistula or a polytetrafluoroethylene (PTFE) graft, sustained increased morbidity and understandable anxiety regarding their dialysis treatments.[1] The creation and subsequent maintenance of hemodialysis access is also expensive. In 1990, Medicare expenditures approximated $383 million for vascular access grafts.[2] Second, the most distal site in the upper extremity still should be selected for vascular access to preserve more proximal sites for future procedures. Because primary autogenous fistulae, irrespective of site, are superior to synthetic grafts in durability, these principles imply that the most distal autogenous fistula should be created before using more proximal synthetic grafts, provided adequate vein is available.

For nondiabetic patients, autogenous forearm options include a snuff-box or cephalic vein (or tributary) to radial artery fistula. The secondary access is usually a synthetic forearm loop graft. Our strategy for the construction of initial dialysis access for diabetic patients differs slightly from this sequence because only 30% of autogenous forearm fistulae in diabetic patients function long enough to initiate cannulation.[3] Therefore, an initial forearm loop

PTFE graft is recommended. The next procedure in the sequence for both diabetic and nondiabetic patients consists of an autogenous upper arm brachiocephalic or transposed basilic vein fistula. An upper arm PTFE graft is the final option because creation of a durable native fistula after a synthetic graft in the upper arm is not usually possible.

CREATION OF TRANSPOSED BASILIC VEIN ARTERIOVENOUS FISTULA
PERIOPERATIVE EVALUATION

The creation of a durable arteriovenous fistula depends on adequate arterial inflow and outflow. Traditionally, the assessment of inflow has been limited to physical examination and demonstration of palmar arch supply through the Allen test. Venous outflow has been assessed in a number of ways. Before the procedure, either as a separate evaluation or in the operating room as the initial maneuver, contrast venography can be performed to delineate the diameter and course of the basilic vein. Although this was routinely performed early in our practice, the lack of anomalies demonstrated by venography has led us to abandon its routine use.

Preoperative ultrasound of the axillo-subclavian venous system is useful in patients with prior central venous catheters or median sternotomy. In addition, patients who have had percutaneously inserted central catheters should also undergo central venous imaging. The increased morbidity of subclinical central venous stenosis ipsilateral to a newly created arteriovenous fistula has been well documented.[4]

SURGICAL TECHNIQUE

Our present technique represents a modification of those previously reported.[5-7] General, regional, or local anesthesia with intravenous sedation has been used with equal success. The planned incision and subdermal tunnel are illustrated in Figure 1. Because the vein must be mobilized to the axillary hairline, the dissection is initiated at the axillary crease. In the event the basilic vein proves anomalous, the procedure can easily be converted to a nonautogenous upper arm fistula.

As illustrated in Figure 2, dissection is continued distally into the antecubital fossa, with preservation of the lateral cutaneous nerve, ensuring maximal length for a tension-free vein within the tunnel. In addition, the brachial artery is easily mobilized through this incision, avoiding a second incision as has been previously described.[5-7] A commercially available tunneling device with interchangeable heads (Subdermal Tunneler, Impra, Inc, Tempe,

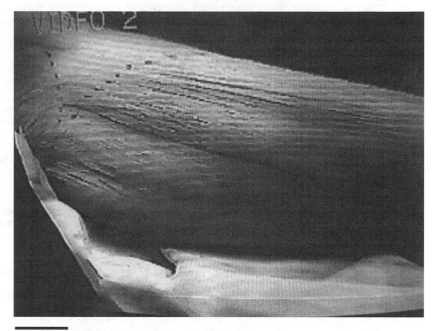

FIGURE 1.
Left upper arm. Dashed line indicates proposed subdermal tunnel location.

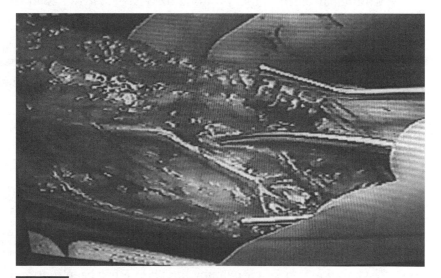

FIGURE 2.
Anticubital exposure of brachiocephalic vein junction. Dissection includes smaller caliber vein for potential anastomosis.

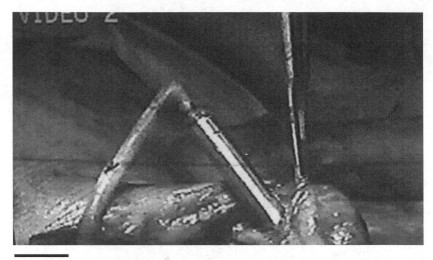

FIGURE 3.
Tunneler in subdermal plain. Vein is distended with saline prior to retraction through tunnel. This prevents axial rotation.

Ariz) is used to create an 8-mm subdermal tunnel. The tunnel is created after the vein is divided at the anticubital fossa, retracted from beneath the lateral cutaneous nerve, and gently distended with heparinized saline solution (5000 U/L) to avoid axial rotation of the transposed vein. Because of the extensive soft tissue dissection, systemic anticoagulation is not used.

Figure 3 illustrates the tunneler emerging from the subdermal location. The tunneling head is exchanged for a 2-mm size, and the vein is tied to the groove of the tunneler without axial rotation. The brachial arteriotomy is limited to 4 mm, and the anastomosis is created with a single continuous 6-0 polypropylene suture. The wound is closed in 2 layers with absorbable suture with subcuticular technique (Fig 4).

RESULTS

In general, the transposed basilic vein arteriovenous fistula (TBAVF) is allowed to mature 2 to 3 weeks before initial cannulation. In patients who have had a prior distal fistula, the basilic vein is usually partially arterialized and may therefore require less time for maturation.

Cumulative primary patency for TBAVF has been reported to be 83% at 1 year, 79% at 1.5 years, and 70% at 8 years.[3,8,9] These results compare favorably with autogenous radiocephalic (67% at 2 years) and brachiocephalic (78% at 1.5 years) fistulae.[3,10]

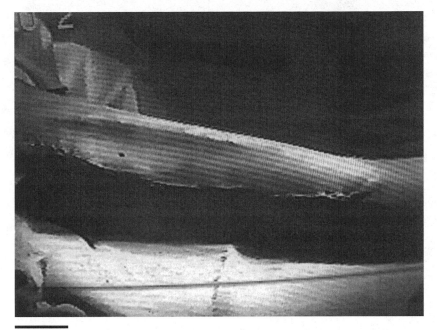

FIGURE 4.
Completed basilic vein transposition fistula. Subcuticular closure.

DISCUSSION

In our experience, the TBAVF represents a durable alternative to nonautogenous conduits for chronic dialysis access. Furthermore, its creation does not preclude future insertion of prosthetic grafts in the same anatomical location should the TBAVF fail.

It is imperative that dialysis personnel are informed that the access is a TBAVF and not a synthetic graft. Otherwise, the so-called "double-puncture" technique may be used with excessive infiltration and loss of the access.

REFERENCES

1. Bay WH, Van Cleef S, Owens M: The hemodialysis access: Preferences and concerns of patients, dialysis nurses, technicians, and physicians. *Am J Nephrol* 18:379-383, 1998.
2. Neumann ME: RAND report: Medicare spent $383 million on placing vascular access grafts in 1990. *Nephrol News Issues* 9:38-39, 1995.
3. Hakaim AG, Nalbandian M, Scott T: Superior maturation and patency of primary brachiocephalic and transposed basilic vein arteriovenous fistulae in patients with diabetes. *J Vasc Surg* 27:154-157, 1998.

4. Cimochowski GE, Worley E, Rutherford WE, et al: Superiority of the internal jugular over subclavian access for temporary hemodialysis. *Nephron* 54:154-156, 1990.

5. Dagher F, Gerber R, Ramos E, et al: The use of basilic vein and brachial artery as an AV fistula for long-term hemodialysis. *J Surg Res* 20:373-376, 1976;.

6. LoGerfo FW, Menzoian JO, Kumaki DJ, et al: Transposed basilic vein brachial arteriovenous fistula. *Arch Surg* 113:1008-1010, 1978.

7. Rivers SP, Scher LA, Sheehan E, et al: Basilic vein transposition: An underused autogenous alternative to prosthetic dialysis angioaccess. *J Vasc Surg* 18:391-397, 1993.

8. Davis JB, Howell CG, Humphries AL Jr: Hemodialysis access: Elevated basilic vein arteriovenous fistula. *J Pediatr Surg* 21:1182-1183, 1986.

9. Dagher FJ: The upper arm AV hemoaccess: Long term follow-up. *J Cardiovasc Surg* 27:447-449, 1986.

10. Mandel SR, Martin PL, Blumoff RL, et al: Vascular access in a university transplant and dialysis program. *Arch Surg* 112:1375-1380, 1977.

CHAPTER 10

Management of the Thrombosed Dialysis-Access Graft

Lewis V. Owens, MD
Vascular Surgery Fellow, Department of Surgery, Division of Vascular Surgery, University of North Carolina at Chapel Hill School of Medicine

Blair A. Keagy, MD
Professor and Chief, Department of Surgery, Division of Vascular Surgery, University of North Carolina at Chapel Hill School of Medicine

William A. Marston, MD
Assistant Professor of Surgery, Department of Surgery, Division of Vascular Surgery, University of North Carolina at Chapel Hill School of Medicine

Access surgery for hemodialysis has seen immense growth and innovation since Kolff created the first practical dialysis machine in 1944.[1] At that time, vascular access for hemodialysis was limited to the treatment of acute renal failure with the placement of temporary metal, glass, or plastic cannulas into arteries and veins. However, with the introduction in the 1960s of the Teflon external arteriovenous shunt by Quinton and colleagues,[2] and the radiocephalic fistula by Brescia and Cimino,[3] hemodialysis for chronic end-stage renal disease (ESRD) became feasible. After these developments, the subcutaneous fistula—either the autogenous radiocephalic type or the prosthetic bridge shunt—became the primary means of permanent hemodialysis access. As our ability to access the circulation has improved, and hemodialysis techniques have been refined, the number of patients eligible for dialysis has increased dramatically. At present, more than 40,000 new cases of ESRD occur each year, and 60% of these patients undergo hemodialysis.[4] As a result, the maintenance of functional vascular access has become an important and challenging problem.

DIALYSIS-GRAFT PATENCY

Prosthetic dialysis grafts are plagued by a high rate of failure (Fig 1). The duration of primary patency for hemodialysis shunts using synthetic graft material has averaged less than 2 years in most reports. Many centers are aggressive in their attempts to construct primary arteriovenous fistulas, because the associated patency rate is significantly better than that with prosthetic shunts. Unfortunately, however, fewer than 50% of patients in most dialysis populations in the United States have veins of sufficient size to construct functional arteriovenous fistulas. The average hemodialysis patient can expect an episode of shunt thrombosis every 12 to 15 months, resulting in numerous procedures to maintain access patency.[5] Access problems are the most common reason for hospital admissions among dialysis patients, accounting for more than $500 million each year in health-care costs.

There have been several novel approaches to improving primary patency of hemodialysis access. Experimental graft materials incorporating stretch- or carbon-coated polytetrafluoroethylene (PTFE) are thought to provide a more stable graft surface with less associated intimal hyperplasia. Mechanical changes in access grafts include the use of tapered grafts to reduce vibration and the creation of a distal hood to minimize blood-flow turbulence.[6, 7]

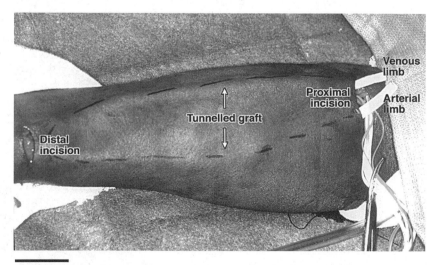

FIGURE 1.
Standard 6-mm PTFE forearm arteriovenous dialysis graft. Distal incision located 2 finger-widths proximal to wrist crease and proximal incision located 1 finger-width distal to elbow crease.

Brachyradiotherapy has been introduced as a way to prevent restenosis after coronary angioplasty, and an experience with this approach with the use of an external beam on dialysis grafts has been reported.[8] Finally, gene therapy directed at factors associated with intimal hyperplasia is an intriguing possibility.[9] Although none of these approaches has yet met with meaningful clinical success, research continues in these potentially important areas.

GRAFT SURVEILLANCE AND PREVENTION

In the dialysis unit, the surgeon can be confronted with a variety of access problems, including access sites that provide insufficient or reduced hemodialysis volume or flow rates. A flow rate of less than 300 mL/min is inadequate for efficient dialysis and may require shunt revision. Skin breakdown overlying an access site often requires graft modification or rerouting, whereas overwhelming infection may respond only to complete removal of a synthetic graft. Pseudoaneurysms often occur at the sites of needle puncture or graft anastomoses and may require surgical revision. Despite the challenges presented by these problems, however, the most common therapeutic dilemma faced by the access surgeon is what to do with an entirely thrombosed PTFE graft.

Once graft thrombosis occurs, access salvage rarely succeeds when viewed from any perspective longer than 3 months. Early detection of access-graft dysfunction and elective surgical revision before thrombosis occurs clearly prolongs access patency. Stenosis at the venous anastomosis is the most common cause of graft dysfunction, but arterial anastomotic and central venous stenosis, as well as intragraft abnormalities, all can contribute to graft failure. The most reliable method for early identification of graft dysfunction has yet to be established. Angiography remains the standard method to document angioaccess lesions, but it is relatively expensive and is associated with modest risks of its own. Elaborate venous-pressure monitoring or the simple observation of elevated venous pressures during dialysis also have been shown to be useful. Recently, we found that surveillance with color-flow duplex imaging (CFDI) appears to be a reliable screening tool in hemodialysis patients.[10]

To explore this we evaluated the efficacy of CFDI versus traditional contrast venography in detecting obstructions in proximal upper extremity venous outflow in patients undergoing hemodialysis. We imaged 60 upper extremities in 42 patients with both CFDI and venography. On the basis of the results, we constructed the decision algorithm presented in Figure 2. We found that CFDI

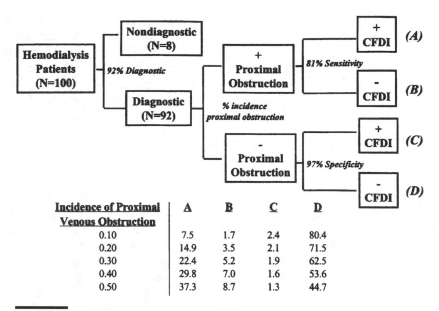

Incidence of Proximal Venous Obstruction	A	B	C	D
0.10	7.5	1.7	2.4	80.4
0.20	14.9	3.5	2.1	71.5
0.30	22.4	5.2	1.9	62.5
0.40	29.8	7.0	1.6	53.6
0.50	37.3	8.7	1.3	44.7

FIGURE 2.
Decision algorithm for color-flow duplex imaging based on diagnostic efficacy and incidence of proximal venous outflow obstruction. *A*, true positive; *B*, false negative. *C*, false positive; *D*, true negative. (Courtesy of Passman MA, Criado E, Farber MA, et al: Efficacy of color flow duplex imaging for proximal upper extremity venous outflow obstruction in hemodialysis patients. *J Vasc Surg* 28:869-875, 1998.)

is an accurate, reliable method to detect such obstructions and should replace contrast venography as the initial imaging study in hemodialysis patients. It remains unclear, however, whether CFDI surveillance in asymptomatic patients will improve long-term patency of hemodialysis access, will be cost-effective, or will be approved for reimbursement by third-party payors.[11]

GRAFT THROMBOSIS

Some authors recommend that thrombosed shunts be abandoned in favor of a new access site. However, a growing number of patients with renal failure require long-term dialysis for 5 to 10 years or longer. If thrombosed shunts are routinely abandoned, many patients will exhaust their desirable upper-extremity shunt sites and will require alternative sites, such as in the leg or chest wall. In at least some of these patients, all available sites may be used eventually, thus prohibiting further hemodialysis. For these reasons, each dialysis site should be preserved for use as long as possible. An optimal protocol for the management of occluded shunts has not been defined, but according to the Clinical Practice Guidelines of the National Kidney Foundation's Dialysis Outcomes Quality Initiative (DOQI), shunts should be salvaged rapidly, and central venous catheters should be avoided.[12] Shunt salvage should be performed with the use of local anesthesia on an outpatient basis whenever possible. Moreover, the initial success and long-term function rates after salvage should be acceptable and cost-effective.

Currently, dialysis graft salvage may be attempted with the use of surgical or percutaneous endovascular techniques. Each has advantages and disadvantages, but both are expensive and result in limited durability of graft function after salvage. As dialysis centers confront potential shifts to capitated reimbursement for services, cost-effective maintenance of dialysis access becomes increasingly important. It is imperative that centers develop protocols for management to allow effective use of manpower and resources and to preserve access sites for optimal patient care.

SURGICAL MANAGEMENT

The surgical approach to salvage of thrombosed dialysis shunts is fairly straightforward, but careful surgical planning is important. In contrast to thrombosis of PTFE graft material, complete thrombosis of an autologous arteriovenous fistula often is not amenable to thrombectomy because of the dramatic inflammatory response evoked by clotting on vascular endothelial cells. Even in prosthetic grafts, thrombectomy alone rarely will be adequate to permit long-term access function. Most thrombectomies must be done in conjunction with some type of formal revision under regional or local anesthesia. The initial incision may be placed at the apex of a loop graft (Fig 3A, site 2), where it is technically easy to gain control of the arterial and venous limbs of the graft and perform a standard thrombectomy with balloon embolectomy catheters. This approach is most successful for the treatment of acute graft thrombosis caused by an episode of sustained hypotension during dialysis or by prolonged shunt compression after decannulation. It does not permit anastomotic revision, however, and is not recommended under most conditions.

The most common cause of graft thrombosis is stenotic intimal hyperplasia at or near the venous anastomosis. This must be considered when planning the incisions for surgical thrombectomy. For a loop forearm graft, exposure through the original incision near the antecubital crease allows complete thrombectomy of the graft while permitting exposure of both the arterial and venous anastomoses (Fig 3A, site 1). Through this incision, the cause of graft failure can be evaluated completely with a shunt angiogram under fluoroscopy. The angiogram should visualize the outflow veins well into the central circulation, to detect any distant venous outflow stenosis (Fig 4). These are important lesions that probably are often overlooked but may contribute to graft malfunction.[13]

For simple, short-segment venous occlusions, patch angioplasty with the use of prosthetic material usually is adequate (Fig 5B). Longer lesions may require a patch extension into the graft or rerouting of the venous anastomosis to another vein. Unfortunately, it often is difficult to find another vein of adequate caliber in the same area. Thus, the best approach is to oversew the graft and leave the venous anastomosis intact while bypassing this area with an additional 6-mm segment of PTFE to an alternative vein site (Fig 5C). This graft should be as short as possible, to allow further revisions if necessary and to preserve venous length for future access procedures. Despite our initial reservations, we have found that extending forearm grafts across the antecubital fossa has produced acceptable results.

Other creative maneuvers to preserve a thrombosed upper-extremity site include developing a new loop around an old loop (Fig 3B, site 3) or placing an arc across the old loop (Fig 3B, site 4).

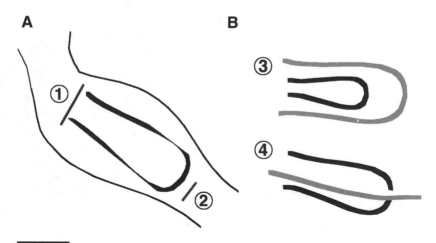

FIGURE 3.
Possible incision sites for revision of a forearm dialysis graft **(A)**: *1*, original incision site; *2*, apex of a loop graft. Options to preserve upper-extremity access sites **(B)**: *3*, new loop around an old loop; *4*, arc across an old loop.

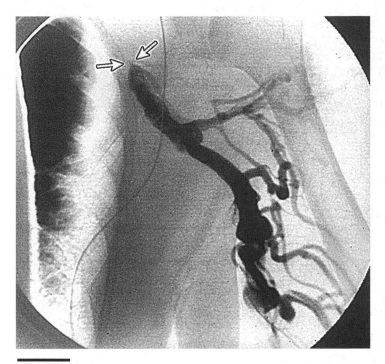

FIGURE 4.
Subclavian vein thrombosis contributing to arm graft failure.

When forearm sites have been depleted, always consider an upper-arm brachial- cephalic or basilic-vein transposition fistula before constructing a synthetic graft in the upper arm. If all upper-extremity sites have been exhausted, the thigh may be used for an end-to-side loop graft (8 mm) between the superficial femoral artery and the saphenous vein. Patency rates for thigh grafts are better than arm sites because of greater fistula flow, but adequate preoperative ankle/brachial pressures should be obtained to reduce the risk of the "arterial steal" phenomenon. Numerous other exotic anastomoses can be carried out to maintain dialysis access, such as an axillo-axillary ("necklace") graft. This graft, relatively easy to perform through an infraclavicular incision, can be useful in some cases of central vein stenosis. The loop graft is placed along the chest wall and is reasonably effective in thin individuals.

As indicated, it is important to recognize central venous outflow obstruction and treat it aggressively to prevent recurrent access-graft thrombosis. To evaluate this problem, we reviewed 158 upper-extremity hemodialysis access procedures performed in

122 patients.[13] Fourteen patients (12%) had a central venous obstruction and associated dialysis-graft dysfunction. All 14 patients had a history of bilateral, temporary, subclavian vein dialysis catheters. Seventeen lesions, including subclavian and internal jugular vein stenoses or occlusions, were treated in these 14 patients. Overall, 21 procedures were performed, including 17 percutaneous transluminal balloon angioplasties (PTAs) with stent

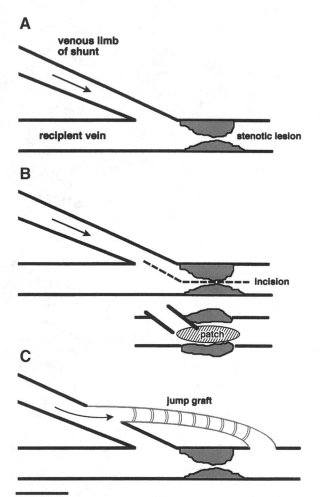

FIGURE 5.
A, Venous limb intimal hyperplasia creating a stenosis and later graft failure. **B,** Correction of short-segment venous occlusion with patch angioplasty using prosthetic material. **C,** Correction of longer-segment venous occlusion with venous bypass using prosthetic material.

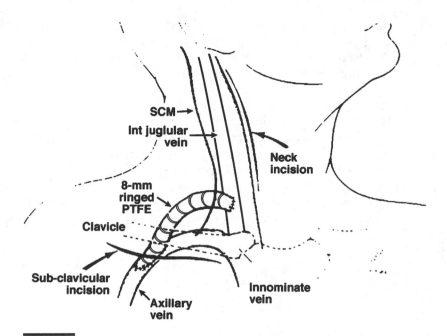

FIGURE 6.
Axillary-internal jugular vein bypass for central venous stenosis using 8-mm ringed PTFE tunneled infraclavicularly.

placement in 13, and either axillary-innominate vein bypass or axillary-internal jugular vein bypass (Fig 6), each in 2 patients. Of the 17 PTAs, 13 (76%) were successful initially, with 80% primary or secondary patency at 6 months. The 4 PTA failures were treated by venous bypasses, which remained patent and provided functional access at 12 months postoperatively. Central vein stenosis is an important cause of dialysis-shunt thrombosis and usually requires complex interventions to ensure future graft patency.

PERCUTANEOUS TECHNIQUES

In recent years, radiographically-guided percutaneous interventions for failing or failed hemodialysis access shunts have become accepted treatment alternatives to traditional surgical management. During these procedures, grafts are accessed in two places along both the arterial and venous limbs using a cross-wire technique (Fig 7). Mechanical thrombectomy using percutaneously placed catheters can be done, pushing the clot into the venous circulation. Numerous devices have been designed to aid in this process and limit clot embolization. Alternatively, pulse-spray thrombolytics — currently, tissue plasminogen activator, or tPA— are given along with balloon or Venturi maceration of the clot. Once the shunt has been cleared by either approach, a shunt angiogram is performed to evaluate the arterial and venous anastomoses as well as the central venous outflow (Fig 8). Stenotic central segments in the axillary, subclavian, or innominate veins that are resistant to balloon angioplasty can be treated with stent placement.

The advantages of endovascular shunt salvage are that it is less invasive than surgical treatment and requires only local anesthesia along with the superior imaging available in angiography suites. Multiple procedures may be performed to maintain access patency without the need for proximal venous surgery. Additionally, as a general rule percutaneous procedures in the interventional radi-

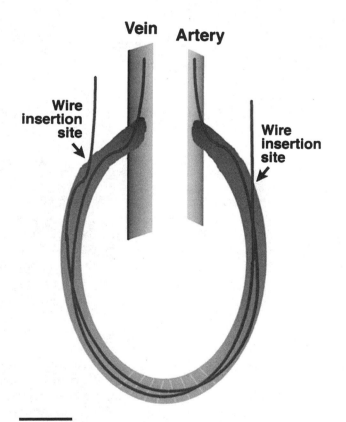

FIGURE 7.
Cross-wire technique to access arterial and venous limbs of a dialysis graft during percutaneous intervention.

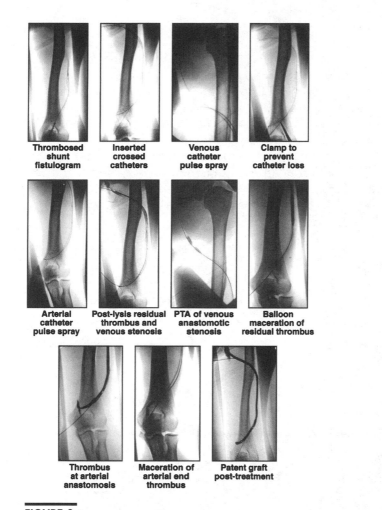

FIGURE 8.
Sequence of percutaneous interventions performed while attempting to excise thrombus from a dialysis graft. (Courtesy of Fumpe D, Durham J, Mann D: Thrombolysis and percutaneous transluminal angioplasty, in Wilson [ed]: *Vascular Access: Principles and Practice.* 3rd ed. St. Louis, Mosby-Year Book, Inc, 1995.

ology suite usually are easier to schedule than surgical thrombectomies in the operating room.

We recently reported the results of a prospective randomized trial comparing the percutaneous approach (mechanical, thrombolytic pulse-spray, or both) with the surgical approach (thrombectomy with patch angioplasty or jump revision of the venous anastomosis).[14] A total of 115 patients with PTFE graft thrombosis were randomized to surgical (n = 56) or endovascular (n = 59) treatment. All patients were treated within 48 hours of diagnosis. The initial success rates were 73% in the percutaneous group and 82% in the surgical (Fig 9). The 3- and 6-month primary patency rates were substantially better in the surgical group than in the endovascular group, but the overall duration of graft function in both groups was disappointing, with only 34% of shunts in the surgical group and 11% in the percutaneous group remaining functional at 6 months. A very significant observation was made about the type of pathology present. The most common finding was a relatively focal venous outflow stenosis, accounting for 55%

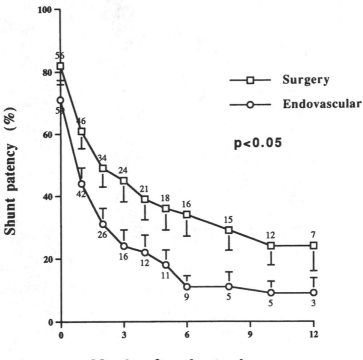

Months after shunt salvage

FIGURE 9.

Primary graft patency rates after surgical versus endovascular salvage of thrombosed shunts. Patency rates differ significantly by the log-rank test ($P < .05$). (Courtesy of Marston WA, Criado E, Jaques PF, et al: Prospective randomized comparison of surgical versus endovascular management of thrombosed dialysis access grafts. *J Vasc Surg* 26:373-380, 1997.)

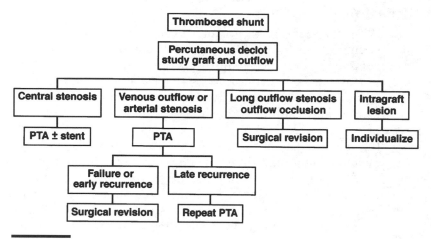

FIGURE 10.
Algorithm of initial approach for acute thrombosis of PTFE dialysis graft.

of cases. These patients fared better when treated surgically, with a 6-month patency rate of 44%. These results emphasize the importance of understanding the nature of the pathology to plan procedures properly. Performing surgical shunt salvage without fluoroscopic guidance will inevitably lead to substandard results in some patients. In this study, the patency rate after a single surgical intervention was significantly better than after a single percutaneous intervention. The long-term success of each technique after multiple, sequential interventions has not been studied in a prospective trial. We conclude that surgical salvage, if optimized by rapid operating-room access, fluoroscopic guidance, and proper patient selection, will yield results that are comparable with the standards established in the DOQI guidelines. The best results, however, may result from the use of fluoroscopy to determine treatment based on the underlying cause of thrombosis.

In the final analysis, percutaneous and surgical techniques are not competitive as much as they are complementary. Future studies should attempt to compare algorithms for treatment using combinations of surgical and percutaneous techniques. Currently, the best outcomes result from multidisciplinary planning, with local preferences and availability of procedure rooms playing a significant role in determining the treatment algorithm. Our approach to the thrombosed PTFE dialysis graft is presented in Figure 10. We believe that this approach maximizes graft patency while minimizing cost, the need for temporary catheters, and patient trauma.

SUMMARY

With the continued, frequent use of prosthetic hemodialysis shunts in the United States, graft thrombosis is likely to remain a common occurrence requiring significant resources to maintain vascular access. As outlined by the DOQI, intensive monitoring of access sites and the elective treatment of those that have significant stenotic lesions or dysfunction should reduce the incidence of thrombosis. Techniques to salvage grafts that already have thrombosed cannot be chosen merely on the basis of cost efficiency. Other important issues need to be considered, including the need for rapid treatment, vein preservation, and long-term function after single or multiple procedures. Perhaps these considerations can be incorporated into prospective studies, in an attempt to develop treatment protocols that will improve the results of prosthetic dialysis grafts and thereby conserve the resources necessary for their maintenance.

REFERENCES

1. Kolff WJ, Berk HTJ, terWelle M, et al: The artificial kidney: A dialyzer with a great area. *Acta Med Scand* 117:121-134, 1944.
2. Quinton WE, Dillard DH, Scribner BH: Cannulation of blood vessels for prolonged hemodialysis. *Trans Am Soc Artif Intern Organs* 6:104-113, 1960.
3. Brescia MJ, Cimino JE, Appel K, et al: Chronic hemodialysis using venipuncture and a surgically created arteriovenous fistula. *N Engl J Med* 275:1089-1092, 1966.
4. United States Renal Data System: Excerpts from United States Renal Data System 1991 annual data report. *Am J Kidney Dis* 18(Suppl 2):1-127, 1991.
5. Port FK: The end-stage renal disease program: Trends over the past 18 years. *Am J Kidney Dis* 20(Suppl 1):3-7, 1992.
6. Fillinger MF, Reinitz ER, Schwartz RA, et al: Beneficial effects of banding on venous intimal-medial hyperplasia in arteriovenous loop grafts. *Am J Surg* 158:87-94, 1989.
7. Fillinger MF, Reinitz ER, Schwartz RA, et al: Graft geometry and venous intimal-medial hyperplasia in arteriovenous loop grafts. *J Vasc Surg* 11:556-566, 1990.
8. Teirstein PS, Massullo V, Jani S, et al: Catheter-based radiotherapy to inhibit restenosis after coronary stenting. *N Engl J Med* 336:1697-1703, 1997.
9. Wilson JM, Birinyi LK, Salomon RN, et al: Implantation of vascular grafts lined with genetically modified endothelial cells. *Science* 244:1344-1346, 1989.
10. Passman MA, Criado E, Farber MA, et al: Efficacy of color flow duplex imaging for proximal upper extremity venous outflow obstruction in hemodialysis patients. *J Vasc Surg* 28:869-875, 1998.

11. Sands J, Young S, Miranda C: The effect of Doppler flow screening studies and elective revisions on dialysis access failure. *ASAIO J* 38:M524-M527, 1992.
12. National Kidney Foundation-Dialysis Outcomes Quality Initiative: NKF DOQI clinical practice guidelines for hemodialysis vascular access. *Am J Kidney Dis* 30(Suppl 3):S150-S191, 1997.
13. Criado E, Marston WA, Jaques PF, et al: Proximal venous outflow obstruction in patients with upper extremity arteriovenous dialysis access. *Ann Vasc Surg* 8:530-535, 1994.
14. Marston WA, Criado E, Jaques PF, et al: Prospective randomized comparison of surgical versus endovascular management of thrombosed dialysis access grafts. *J Vasc Surg* 26:373-380, 1997.

CHAPTER 11

Hemodynamic Basis for the Diagnosis and Treatment of Angioaccess-induced Steal Syndrome

Christopher L. Wixon, MD
Clinical Resident, University of Arizona, University Medical Center, Tucson

Joseph L. Mills, Sr, MD
Professor of Surgery, University of Arizona, Chief, Section of Vascular Surgery, University Medical Center, Tucson

Complications related to hemodialysis access surgery may evoke a variety of reactions including denial, consternation, and occasionally anger. The development of ischemic steal syndrome is no exception. The surgeon struggles with the dilemma created by the seemingly conflicting objectives of maintaining fistula patency and restoring peripheral perfusion. Unfortunately, surgical interventions based on increasing fistula resistance (banding or lengthening) continue to disappoint both the surgeon and patient because such approaches frequently eventuate in either fistula thrombosis or inadequate resolution of ischemic symptoms. However, the recently described distal revascularization–interval ligation (DRIL) procedure resolves the dilemma by providing not only reliable relief of ischemic symptoms, but also excellent preservation of fistula patency.[1] This chapter clearly defines the clinical syndrome and provides a physiologic treatment algorithm for management of ischemic steal related to hemodialysis access procedures.

DEFINING THE ISCHEMIC STEAL SYNDROME

During the last decade, the number of persons with renal failure has nearly doubled. The current estimate of patients on hemodialysis exceeds 180,000, and this patient population is expected to continue to grow at an annual rate of 7% to 9%.[2] For these patients, complications related to vascular access remain the most common cause of morbidity and mortality. Annual expenditures for access-related complications exceed $1 billion.[2] In 1995, these issues prompted the National Kidney Foundation to establish the Dialysis Outcome Quality Initiative, which focuses on improving outcome and survival of patients with end-stage renal disease.[3] These guidelines firmly endorse attempts at the establishment of an autogenous hemodialysis access and establish a goal of 40% to 50% prevalence of autogenous fistulae among all hemodialysis patients. To meet these guidelines at the University of Arizona, it has become necessary to extend the application of autogenous fistulae to older patients, diabetic patients, and patients in whom previous access procedures have been performed. As a result of this practice, we have recently noted an increased incidence of ischemic steal syndrome.

Clinically significant distal extremity ischemia occurs in 1.6% to 8% of all individuals with a functioning dialysis shunt.[4-11] Risk factors include female sex, age greater than 60 years, diabetes, multiple operations on the same limb, the construction of an autogenous fistula, and the use of the brachial artery as the donor vessel.[8,10,11]

Symptoms associated with the ischemic steal syndrome present over a broad spectrum, ranging from vague neurosensory deficits (frequently mistaken for diabetic neuropathy) to ischemic rest pain or tissue loss. In severe cases, patients have permanent neuromotor changes. Physical examination often reveals diminished peripheral pulses, pallor, weakness, or muscle wasting. Because of

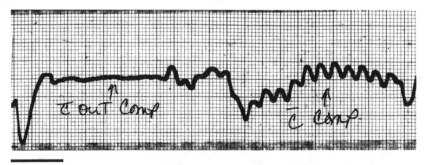

FIGURE 1.
Digital photoplethysmographic (PPG) waveform tracings in a patient with ischemic steal syndrome after placement of an arteriovenous fistula. When the fistula is patent, the waveforms are monophasic, but regain normal pulsatility when the fistula is compressed.

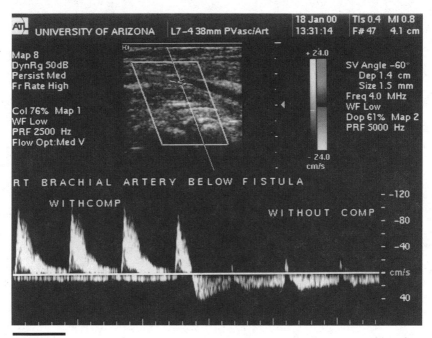

FIGURE 2.
Duplex examination of the brachial artery just distal to an end-side anastomosis of the cephalic vein and the brachial artery. Without compression **(right)**, there is a brief interval of antegrade flow followed by a long interval of retrograde flow during diastole. Compression of the fistula **(left)** restores normal brachial artery waveforms.

the nonspecificity of many of these signs and symptoms, the physician must maintain a high index of suspicion when treating patients with a functioning arteriovenous fistula.

Definitive diagnostic testing can be performed noninvasively by comparing digital photoplethysmographic (PPG) waveforms with and without fistula compression (Fig 1). Although digital perfusion pressures and plethysmographic waveform amplitudes are normally reduced distal to a patent fistula, the waveforms should retain their normal contour.[12,13] Most patients with significant steal have monophasic, or flat, digital waveforms that normalize or significantly improve with manual compression of the fistula.

Although duplex examination is an important adjunct to physiologic testing, duplex alone is not sufficient to establish the diagnosis. We have detected retrograde blood flow in the artery just distal to the fistula in several patients in whom ischemic symptoms could not be elicited (Fig 2). This pattern is most commonly observed in the Cimino fistula (radial artery to cephalic vein), but has likewise been observed at the level of the brachial artery. That is, not only does the fistula consume the antegrade flow in the artery at the level of the fistula, but it also consumes a portion of the collateral blood flow by way of retrograde flow in the artery distal to the fistula. Nevertheless, identification of retrograde blood flow in the artery distal to the fistula is not sufficient to make the diagnosis of the ischemic steal syndrome. Rather, the diagnosis remains a clinical one, supplemented by the PPG digital waveform studies, with and without fistula compression.

FISTULA PHYSIOLOGY

Effective treatment of patients with ischemic steal syndrome demands a thorough understanding of the hemodynamics associated with a patent arteriovenous fistula. These hemodynamics have interested surgeons and physiologists since William Hunter's description of the *aneurysm varix* in 1764.[14] However, a true physiologic understanding did not evolve until the comprehensive work by Emile Holman,[15,16] Mont Reid,[17] and others.[18] These studies hold true to the spirit of Hunterian curiosity and serve as classic examples of surgical research.

The basic components of an arteriovenous fistula (Fig 3) include a common inflow (donor artery) and outflow conduit (outflow vein); a low-flow, high-resistance connection (the peripheral vascular bed); a high-flow, low-resistance connection (the fistula); and a parallel set of inflow and outflow conduits (the arterial and venous collaterals). The patterns of pressure and flow in the fistula and peripheral vascular bed are determined by the resistances of each component.

The creation of an arteriovenous fistula has several important effects on the flow patterns of the arterial and venous circulation. Obviously, in all circumstances, the direction of blood flow in the proximal artery remains toward the periphery (centrifugal), and the direction of blood flow in the proximal vein remains toward the heart (centripetal). Likewise, the direction of blood flow in the arterial and venous collaterals remains predictable, with arterial collateral flow directed peripherally and venous collateral flow directed centrally. The direction of blood flow in the artery distal to the fistula is variable, however, and may be antegrade, retrograde, or bidirectional depending on the pressure gradients of the proximal artery, the arterial collaterals, the fistula, and the peripheral vascular bed.[18]

Theoretically, the presence of a large arteriovenous fistula always results in reduced perfusion to more peripheral tissues. This is evidenced by the fact that the perfusion pressure is always

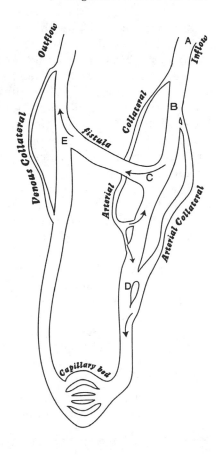

FIGURE 3.

Basic components of an arteriovenous fistula. *Arrows* represent direction of blood flow. Note that blood flow in the artery just distal to the fistula may be antegrade, retrograde, or both. (Courtesy of Wixon CL, Mills JL, Berman SS: Distal revascularization–internal ligation for maintenance of dialysis access and restoration of distal reperfusion in ischemic steal syndrome. *Semin Vasc Surg* 13:77-82, 2000.)

lower distal to an arteriovenous fistula.[19] Under usual circumstances, arterial collaterals and compensatory peripheral vasodilatation are sufficient to maintain peripheral perfusion at adequate levels. *The consequences of the fistula blood flow become significant only if distal arterial perfusion pressure is insufficient to satisfy peripheral metabolic requirements.*

TREATING THE ISCHEMIC STEAL SYNDROME

The natural history of the ischemic steal syndrome was evaluated by Lazarides et al.[10] They demonstrated that in 80% of patients who have symptoms acutely after the establishment of an arteriovenous fistula, the systolic pressure index (SPI, finger pressure/systemic pressure) improved over 2 to 4 months without surgical intervention. Indeed, distal ischemia serves as a potent stimulus for the development of a rich collateral network that partially compensates for the diminished peripheral perfusion pressure. As such, we tend to observe patients with mild early steal syndrome after arteriovenous access procedures. We reserve surgical intervention for patients with severe ischemia and patients who fail to improve based on noninvasive, physiologic testing (SPI). In contradistinction, symptoms that occur late (> 30 days after placement of the fistula) are frequently progressive and tend not to resolve with conservative therapy. These patients require identification and surgical intervention to prevent permanent ischemic neuropathy.

We have identified 3 clinical scenarios in which significant ischemic steal syndrome occurs: steal that occurs on hemodialysis, steal caused by an inflow stenosis, and steal resulting from discordant fistula/peripheral vascular resistance. Because these differ in etiology and treatment, each presentation is discussed independently.

STEAL DURING HEMODIALYSIS

A somewhat confusing situation arises in a small subset of patients who have transient ischemic symptoms only while undergoing hemodialysis. In one recent patient, symptoms were so severe that dialysis could not be continued through her fistula. Curiously, the symptoms recurred with equal intensity when dialysis was initiated using a temporary internal jugular catheter. Review of her dialysis record showed a 20 mm Hg decrease in mean arterial pressure as a result of reduced myocardial preload. We asked the patient to not take her antihypertensive medicine the following morning and again performed dialysis through her temporary internal jugular catheter. Her mean arterial pressure remained greater than 65 mm Hg, and the steal symptoms were significantly improved.

This example illustrates the common misconception that this phenomenon is secondary to an increased brachial shunt fraction (fistula blood flow/brachial artery blood flow) on dialysis. However, because the high-capacitance outflow vein quickly dampens the pressure gradient generated by the dialysis pump, it is unlikely that fistula shunt fractions are significantly augmented during dialysis. Rather, these patients have a significant reduction in systemic blood pressure caused by hypovolemia and a resultant diminished myocardial preload. The relative reduction in proximal perfusion pressure exceeds compensatory mechanisms of the peripheral vascular bed and establishes a temporary condition of global distal ischemia. These symptoms slowly resolve on cessation of dialysis. Therefore, for patients who have mild to moderate ischemic symptoms only while on hemodialysis, our first line of therapy is to hold antihypertensive medicines on the morning of dialysis. In our experience, this has been successful in alleviating, or partially alleviating, ischemic symptoms in the majority of patients. With this in mind, therapies directed at alleviating symptoms by reducing dialysis pump flow rates remain dubious.

STEAL CAUSED BY AN INFLOW LESION

The presence of a proximal inflow stenosis contributes to the steal syndrome in approximately 20% to 30% of patients who have distal extremity ischemia.[8,9,11] Therefore, selective arteriography of the donor artery remains a critical portion of the evaluation before embarking on surgical revision to correct symptomatic steal syndrome. It is also important to consider that traditional anatomical predictors of hemodynamic significance may not apply to lesions proximal to an arteriovenous fistula. The increased flow velocity in the proximal artery contributes to an increased viscosity constant. Examining Poiseuille's law,

$$P = 8L\eta V/r^2$$

where L is the length of stenosis, η is the viscosity constant of blood, V is the mean velocity of blood flow across the stenosis, and r is the radius of stenosis, we see that the increased viscosity constant and increased mean velocity in the proximal artery contribute to an increased pressure gradient across a lesion. Therefore, traditional predictors of significance, based only on percent stenosis, may fail to identify hemodynamically significant lesions. It is therefore recommended that hemodynamic significance be assessed by determination of pressure gradients across all suspicious lesions. These may then be corrected by catheter-based or surgical means.

STEAL CAUSED BY DISCORDANT VASCULAR RESISTANCE

The most commonly occurring and challenging form of ischemic steal syndrome is that caused by discordant vascular resistance. Successful treatment mandates that the surgeon recognize the existing disparity between the resistances of the peripheral circulation and the fistula. For many years, the most commonly suggested procedures to treat steal syndrome were banding, plicating, or lengthening the fistula so as to increase fistula resistance and decrease fistula blood flow. To gauge the precise degree of narrowing such that adequate peripheral perfusion is restored, investigators have used digital PPG testing during banding procedures.[11,20] Despite these physiologic measures, however, review of clinical series in which this technique has been used demonstrates inconsistent restoration of distal perfusion and high rates of fistula thrombosis.[9,11]

The inability to reconcile the seemingly competing hemodynamic effect of the fistula and the metabolic demand of the distal circulation was studied by Schanzer et al[1] in 1988. Although these authors also recognized that the ischemic steal syndrome resulted from a discordant relationship between the resistance in the fistula and the resistance in the periphery, they suggested solving the equation from the side of the peripheral circulation. Schanzer astutely recognized a potential mechanism of inadequate peripheral circulation resulted from a poorly formed arterial collateral network. In an attempt to reduce the resistance in the peripheral circuit, a bypass (in essence, a low-resistance collateral) was created between the artery proximal to the fistula and the artery distal to the fistula. This reduced the resistance ratio between the peripheral circulation and the fistula, reduced the brachial shunt fraction, and directed a greater proportion of blood flow toward the periphery. To prevent retrograde flow up the native artery distal to the fistula, the artery distal to the fistula was ligated (Fig 4).

From a technical standpoint, several points deserve emphasis. At the time of reconstruction, the location of the proximal bypass anastomosis in relation to the arterial pressure sink of the fistula is of critical importance. Although previously described, the significance of the arterial pressure sink has been poorly recognized. It exists secondary to the large capacitance in the outflow veins of the fistula, causing the pressure on the venous side of a fistula to fall off quickly (the pressure on the venous side of the fistula approximates the central venous pressure within 1 cm of the anastomosis). Because the systemic to venous pressure gradient must exist in a continuum, a pressure sink necessarily exists on the arterial side of the fistula (Fig 5).

In our experience, locating the origin of the bypass greater than 3 cm proximal to the origin of the fistula appears to be sufficient and conveniently avoids the need to approach the artery through a reoperative field. In essence, the interposing segment of artery distal to the bypass origin, but proximal to the fistula origin, serves functionally to lengthen the fistula with a low-capacitance, low-resistance conduit. The net benefit removes the origin of the bypass from the "pressure sink" region near the fistula origin. Although the reversed saphenous vein remains our bypass conduit of choice, there can be little logic to the argument that it is necessary to use a segment of reversed vein that contains a competent valve to prevent retrograde flow up the bypass.

Still, of unclear consequence, are the collaterals around the ligated segment of the native brachial artery. Arteriovenous fistula is the most potent hemodynamic stimulus for collateral development,[21] and we have observed collateral networks of remarkable proportion after fistula placement (Fig 6). Some have advocated ligating these branches at the time of the DRIL procedure, arguing that the augmented pressure in the more distal artery could serve

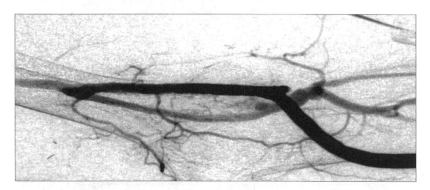

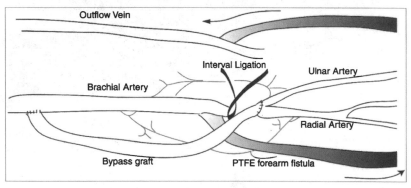

FIGURE 4.
Angiographic and diagrammatic depiction of the distal revascularization–interval ligation (DRIL) procedure. The origin of the bypass should be located sufficiently proximal to the fistula origin to avoid the "pressure sink" region created by the low-resistance fistula.

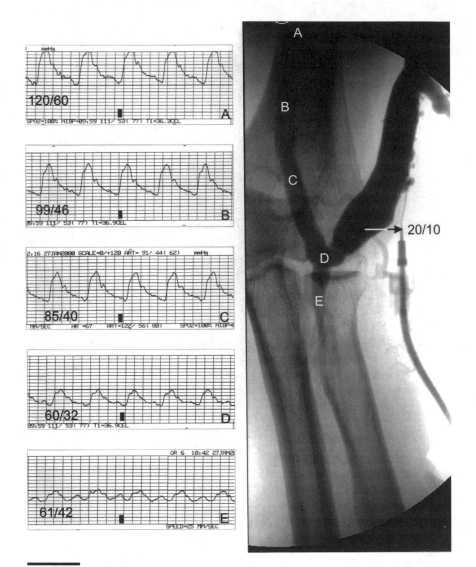

FIGURE 5.
Defining the "pressure sink" of an arteriovenous fistula. Brachial artery pressure tracings were acquired using an end-hole catheter at variable distances from the fistula origin.

to reflux flow back into the segment of artery that leads to the fistula. In our experience, this has not been necessary.

Finally, as previously discussed, a fraction of patients exists in whom there is significant retrograde flow in the artery distal to the fistula.[6,18] That is, in addition to diverting the entire blood flow of

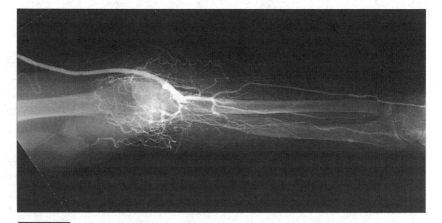

FIGURE 6.
Intraoperative arteriogram of the brachial artery bypass demonstrates a rich collateral network around the origin of the fistula.

the more proximal donor artery, the fistula also consumes flow from the arterial collateral network through retrograde flow up the artery distal to the fistula. In this situation, ligating the artery just distal to the fistula would theoretically eliminate the retrograde flow and improve the peripheral perfusion pressure. Although this has been demonstrated in an animal model,[18] its clinical utility remains uncertain. We have witnessed only modest improvement in peripheral perfusion pressures when ligation is performed without concomitant bypass. As such, we have applied it only in cases of steal caused by an end-side Cimino fistula at the wrist.

SURGICAL RESULTS

Ten years have passed since Schanzer's first description of the operation that has since been termed the DRIL procedure, named for its 2 essential components. Application of this technique in a recent series of 21 patients demonstrated uniform resolution of ischemic symptoms.[8] Patency of the bypass graft was 100% at a mean of 18 months (life-table analysis), and fistula patency was 94% at a mean of 18 months (life-table analysis). There were no major amputations in any of the patients in that report.

CONCLUSIONS

Although the creation of a proximal arteriovenous fistula always reduces the perfusion pressure of the distal vascular bed, normal compensatory mechanisms—increased collateral circulation, decreased peripheral vascular resistance—are usually sufficient to maintain normal perfusion. However, when arteriovenous fistula flow exceeds these compensatory mechanisms, distal ischemia occurs.

The development of ischemic steal syndrome remains an important complication after creation of an arteriovenous fistula. Before the description of the DRIL procedure, attempts at fistula banding frequently failed to correct the distal ischemia or resulted in fistula thrombosis. Because available treatment options were poor, there was a general reluctance for physicians to fully recognize the syndrome. In many centers this reluctance persists, as ongoing attempts at fistula banding continue to disappoint both the patient and the surgeon. The innovative design of the DRIL procedure provides a unique and reliable means to reestablish distal perfusion without compromising the patency of the fistula and is strongly recommended as the procedure of choice in ischemic steal syndrome.

REFERENCES

1. Schanzer H, Schwartz M, Harrington E, et al: Treatment of ischemia due to "steal" by arteriovenous fistula with distal artery ligation and revascularization. *J Vasc Surg* 7:770-773, 1988.
2. United States Renal Data System: The economic cost of ESRD, vascular access procedures, and Medicare spending for alternative modalities of treatment. *Am J Kidney Dis* 30(2 suppl 1):S160-S177, 1997.
3. NKF-DOQI *Clinical Practice Guidelines for Vascular Access*. New York, National Kidney Foundation, 1997.
4. Haimov M, Baez H, Neff M, et al: Complications of arteriovenous fistulas for hemodialysis. *Arch Surg* 110:708-712, 1975.
5. Zibari GB, Rohr MD, Landreneau MD, et al: Complications from permanent hemodialysis access. *Surgery* 104:681-686, 1988.
6. Kwun KB, Schanzer H, Finkler N, et al: Hemodynamic evaluation of vascular angioaccess procedures for hemodialysis. *Vasc Surg* 13:170-177, 1979.
7. Ballard J, Blunt TJ, Malone J: Major complications of angioaccess surgery. *Am J Surg* 164:229-232, 1992.
8. Berman SS, Gentile AT, Glickman MH, et al: Distal revascularization-interval ligation for limb salvage and maintenance of dialysis access in ischemic steal syndrome. *J Vasc Surg* 26:393-404, 1997.
9. Morsy AH, Kulbaski M, Chen C, et al: Incidence and characteristics of patients with ischemia after hemodialysis access procedure. *J Surg Res* 74:8-10, 1998.
10. Lazarides MK, Staamos DN, Panagopoulos GN, et al: Indications for surgical treatment of angioaccess-induced arterial "steal." *J Am Coll Surg* 187:421-426, 1998.
11. DeCaprio JD, Valentine RJ, Kakish MB, et al: Steal syndrome complicating hemodialysis access. *Cardiovasc Surg* 5:648-653, 1997.

12. Strandness DE Jr, Gibbons GE, Bell JW: Mercury strain gauge plethysmography: Evaluation of patients with acquired arteriovenous fistulas. *Arch Surg* 85:215, 1962.

13. Bussell JA, Stevens LE, Weaver DH, et al: Advantages of surgical arteriovenous fistulas for hemodialysis. *Arch Surg* 102:359, 1971.

14. Hunter W: Further observations upon a particular species of aneurysm. *Med Observ Inq* 2:390, 1764.

15. Holman E: *Arteriovenous Aneurysm: Abnormal Communication Between the Arterial and Venous Circulations.* New York, Macmillan, 1937.

16. Holman E: The anatomic and physiologic effects of an arteriovenous fistula. *Surgery* 8:362, 1940.

17. Reid MR, McGuire J: Arteriovenous aneurysms. *Ann Surg* 108:643, 1938.

18. Ingebrigtsen R, When PS: Local blood pressure and direction of flow in experimental arterio-venous fistula. *Acta Chir Scandinav* 120:142-150, 1960.

19. Schenk WG Jr, Martin JW, Leslie MB, et al: The regional hemodynamics of chronic experimental arteriovenous fistulas. *Surg Gynecol Obsstet* 110:44, 1960.

20. Shemesh D, Mabjeesh NJ, Abramowitz HB: Management of dialysis access–associated steal syndrome: Use of intraperative duplex ultrasound scanning for optimal flow reduction. *J Vasc Surg* 30:193-195, 1999.

21. Reid MR: Studies on abnormal arteriovenous communications, acquired and congenital. *Arch Surg* 10:601, 1925.

CHAPTER 12

Impact of Graft Surveillance on Longevity of Vascular Access Sites

Samuel E. Wilson, MD
Professor and Chair, Department of Surgery, University of California, Irvine

Michael A. Peck, MD
Senior Resident in General Surgery, Department of Surgery, University of California, Irvine

Since the introduction of extracorporeal dialysis of blood by Kolff et al[1] in 1944, maintenance of patent vascular access sites has been a constant struggle for physicians caring for patients with end-stage renal disease (ESRD). Chronic hemodialysis patients on the average undergo revision of a thrombosed graft, implantation of a new graft, or placement of a temporary central venous catheter about once a year. Revisions for infection and thrombosis are less frequent by one quarter and one half, respectively, for patients with functioning autogenous arteriovenous (AV) fistulas. Percutaneous central venous catheters for dialysis fail more frequently than grafts.[2] The most common cause of access failure is thrombosis, which is usually the result of decreased conduit flow secondary to stenotic lesions in outflow veins.[3] Although highly accurate in definition, angiography has not been routinely used to diagnose dialysis access stenosis, probably because it is invasive, expensive, and inconvenient. Occasionally, noninvasive studies have been advocated to detect stenotic lesions with the expectation that subsequent surgical correction before thrombosis would prolong longevity of the access site. The 1997 National Kidney Foundation-Dialysis Outcomes Quality Initiative (NKI-DOOI) guidelines have renewed interest in this approach and are examined in this chapter. Surgical revision after graft failure is the usual course of action.

CURRENT PATENCY RATES

Data from experienced vascular surgeons and established dialysis centers show primary patency rates for AV bridge grafts to be just under 50%. For example, Schuman et al,[4] after analyzing 632 patients who had polytetrafluoroethylene (PTFE) grafts, found the primary patency to be 44% at 1 year. In the prospective study of Cinat et al,[5] the primary patency was 43% at 1 year. Kennedy et al[6] calculated a 37% overall graft survival at 2 years based on medical records for 1477 northern New England hemodialysis patients. Secondary patency rates for PTFE grafts are considerably higher; 85% at 1 year for Schuman's patients and 64% in Cinat's report.[4,5] It can be concluded from this clinical information that thrombosis within the first year after implantation of a new graft is to be expected. Secondary intervention can significantly prolong function. Thus, it would seem reasonable to presume that surveillance either by anatomical imaging or physiological tests, which would detect abnormalities in form or function before graft thrombosis, would allow earlier and more successful intervention, leading to prolonged patency. Several surgical groups have analyzed their patients for risk factors that would predict failure of the dialysis access graft. A regression analysis by Hodges et al[7] of patient risk factors in 236 PTFE grafts showed that a history of a previously unsalvageable PTFE graft was the only significant risk factor for failure of a subsequent PTFE graft.

The National Kidney Foundation has embraced the philosophy of graft surveillance, rightly concerned that "hemodialysis access failure is the most frequent cause of hospitalization among ESRD patients." A Vascular Access Work Group has been formed to provide guidelines derived from evidence-based criteria that would assist surgeons who establish vascular access sites. These guidelines, published as the "NKF-DOQI Practice Guidelines for Vascular Access," have 2 concluding recommendations: first, increase the use of autogenous AV fistulas and second, detect access dysfunction before access thrombosis.[8] The latter recommendations are based on the belief that an "aggressive policy for monitoring AV-graft patency extends graft life and minimizes graft thrombosis." Although the data reviewed in the NKF-DOQI article relate decrease in blood flow to venous outflow stenosis, there is no substantial evidence cited that prophylactic correction of stenotic areas of the venous runoff segment prolongs graft patency.

Nevertheless, the authors believe that intervention with percutaneous transluminal angioplasty or a surgical revision to correct stenosis "dramatically reduces the rate of AV graft thrombosis and loss." Monitoring is therefore recommended at monthly intervals, including physical examination, Doppler study, dynamic or static venous pressures, and calculation of recirculation values using blood urea concentrations. As the NKF-DOQI Work Group has noted, detection of anatomical stenosis without concomitant measurement of venous pressure or recirculation is probably not helpful.

SITE SELECTION

The success of an autogenous fistula for hemodialysis begins with preoperative selection of optimal veins and arteries, as well as assurance of an adequate venous outflow. The increased use of synthetic bridge grafts in the United States is a likely consequence of a higher early failure rate for fistulas than for grafts, as well as a preference by dialysis personnel for easy puncture. Silva et al[9] has used duplex ultrasound and found more than 60% of arteries and veins in the upper extremity are suitable for AV fistulas. They report a decrease in early failure rate of fistulas from 36% to 8.3% when using preoperative duplex. The predictive role of color Doppler ultrasonography in determining the success of PTFE dialysis access grafts is reported by Koksoy et al.[10] They demonstrate lower preoperative and postoperative brachial artery flow rates in patients whose grafts later thrombose. Preoperative venous duplex examination has also been shown to enhance the durability of bridging grafts in patients with clinical evidence of suboptimal venous runoff. Wladis et al[11] achieved an advantage in graft patency when Doppler studies showed continuity between the venous anastomosis and the central venous system. Doppler studies may not be necessary preoperatively for venous mapping in all patients but are very helpful if veins are not readily detectable and if there are risk factors for axillo-subclavian venous thrombosis such as prolonged central venous catheterization.

PREDICTION OF ACCESS FAILURE

Doppler ultrasound provides both anatomical visualization of a dialysis fistula or graft, including the venous runoff, and certain blood flow measurements derived from velocity. It is reasonable then to expect that a noninvasive test such as duplex ultrasound will assist in predicting impending dialysis access failure. The optimal surveillance interval would depend on ability to predict impending access failure and the cost efficacy of repeat testing.

Strauch et al[12] found that 57% of the patients with venous stenosis greater than 50% by Doppler ultrasound progressed to thrombosis within 6 months as compared with 9.5% of the patients with 30% to 50% stenosis. Sands et al[13] determined that more than 90% of PTFE grafts with flow rates of less than 800 mL/min by ultrasound developed thrombosis within 6 months. Although the data from these two studies were very promising, the trials were not randomized.

In a prospective randomized trial, Lumsden et al[14] used Doppler to discover greater than 50% stenosis in functioning PTFE grafts and then confirmed the findings with angiograms. No improvement was found in patency of PTFE grafts at 12 months in grafts randomly assigned to duplex surveillance and prophylactic angioplasty for stenosis greater than 50%. Control patients had the same degree of stenosis but no intervention. Intervention for anatomical abnormality alone does not seem to prolong graft patency. However, the evidence suggests that Doppler studies of stenoses are likely to become a significant part of dialysis access surveillance but need to be correlated with dialysis function.

The hemodialysis center serves as a convenient and cost-effective laboratory for the surveillance of vascular access grafts. Palpation of the graft should reveal a continuous thrill throughout the graft. A strong pulsatile flow through the graft suggests venous stenosis, and imaging of the graft may be indicated.

VENOUS RETURN PRESSURE

Venous pressure monitoring is based on the premise that resistance to flow increases as stenosis from intimal hyperplasia develops in the venous outflow tract. This is detected as an increased pressure measured in the access proximal to the stenosis. Dynamic venous pressure monitoring was shown to be a reliable method of detecting fistula stenosis in a prospective trial by Schwab et al.[3] Pressures greater than 150 mm Hg at flow rates of 200 to 225 mL/min were considered to be significantly elevated. Eighty-six percent of patients subsequently studied by angiography had venous stenosis of greater than 50%. In contrast, only 7% of grafts with normal pressure measurements had significant stenoses. Using this venous dialysis pressure protocol, there was an 86% sensitivity and a 93% specificity in detecting venous stenosis. The thrombosis rate per patient-year in patients with elevated venous pressures who underwent elective graft revision was comparable to that of patients with normal venous pressures. In contrast, the rate of thrombosis was 10 times greater when venous pressures were elevated but patients refused graft revision. Static venous pressure monitoring corrects for resistance in dialysis tubing and needles that contributes significantly to the venous pressure measured during hemodialysis. The NKF-DOQI guidelines currently recommend dynamic or static pressure monitoring in all dialysis patients as a means to detect outflow stenoses. Both methods have similar sensitivity and specificity, and are the least expensive form of graft surveillance. Dynamic pressures should be obtained weekly, with an increasing trend during a 3-week period suggesting venous stenosis. The greatest drawback to this type of monitoring is the need to standardize tubing and needles. Stenoses tend to occur more centrally in fistulas than in grafts. As a result, collateral veins develop that drain an AV fistula. For this reason, marked increases in pressure do not occur, and indirect pressure measurements do not accurately predict impending fistula failure.[8]

Evidence suggests that a trend of decreasing flow in an access graft is predictive of worsening venous stenosis. The NKF-DOQI guidelines recommend at least monthly monitoring. There are several methods for measuring flow in a dialysis access. Doppler flow, ultrasound transit, and magnetic resonance flow are the most common. Expense often limits the frequency of use of Doppler studies and magnetic resonance. Furthermore, it is difficult to perform these tests during dialysis sessions. Variability in the examiner and equipment diminish the reliability of Doppler results. Access flow is able to be monitored by indicator dilution techniques during hemodialysis sessions. Results are comparable to Doppler ultrasound. Depner et al[15] reported a 77% rate of failure in grafts with baseline flow of less than 600 mL/min over 6 months. Sands[13] found that patients receiving monthly access flow monitoring had decreased thrombosis rates for both fistulas and grafts compared with patients receiving static venous pressure monitoring. The mean of flow rates as determined by Doppler study in the last examination preceding graft thrombosis in a study by Shackelton et al[16] was 417 mL/min.

Monitoring at monthly intervals, which may include physical examination, Doppler study, dynamic or static venous pressures, and calculation of recirculation using blood urea concentrations, is recommended by the DOQI guidelines. The question that arises is, how should such results be applied to ESRD patients in a clinical setting? When should angioplasty or surgical revision be recommended? It is important to note, as the NKF-DOQI Work Group did, that the detection of anatomical stenosis without concomitant measurement of venous pressure or recirculation is probably not helpful. Cinat et al[5] prospectively evaluated graft surveillance techniques to determine their usefulness in predicting PTFE graft patency. Neither venous pressures nor recirculation values were significant in predicting graft failure, although a trend toward increased venous line pressure occurred over time in grafts that failed. No absolute value or percent increase in venous line pressure predicted failure. Blood flow rates during dialysis in grafts that failed averaged 368 ± 34 mL/min compared with 375 ± 24 mL/min in grafts that remained patent throughout the study. The difference was not statistically significant. These and other studies suggest that more accurate physiologic determinants are needed to predict graft failure and that a trend of rising venous line pressures may be the only practical method.

The ultimate goal of achieving longer-lasting hemodialysis access is realistic although not straightforward. The hemodynamic changes imposed on the circulatory system when arteries and veins are directly anastomosed or connected via bridging synthetic grafts produce the condition that gives rise to venous stenosis. The NKF-DOQI guidelines for graft surveillance are a largely evidence-based protocol for improving graft and fistula patency that vascular surgeons and nephrologists should attempt to implement in an effort to improve access patency rates. At the same time, they should be keeping accurate outcome data to assess the usefulness of such surveillance. Percutaneous transluminal angioplasty of anatomical lesions is expensive and unproven; vascular surgeons practical and more convenient for the patient to revise a venous outflow stenosis by patch angioplasty or extension segment while the graft is still functioning and without interrupting dialysis.

We recommend a collaborative effort between the vascular surgeon and dialysis staff that is aimed at optimizing and standardizing graft surveillance. The goal should be improved overall graft patency achieved by predicting which grafts are likely to fail and intervening with graft revision before thrombosis. Patients with chronic renal insufficiency should be referred to the vascular surgeon as early as possible to allow time for the creation and maturation of an autogenous radial artery to cephalic vein fistula. Once a patient is receiving chronic hemodialysis, the dialysis unit should record dynamic line pressure measurements by a standardized method according to dialyzer type on a monthly basis. If a trend of increasing pressures is detected, or if there is abnormal blood flow or recirculation, a duplex scan of the graft should be obtained, looking for hemodynamically significant venous stenosis. An angiogram may be obtained once significant stenosis is detected to aid in determining the method of correction. One imaging study, duplex or angiogram, may be sufficient. The intervention should be planned for a day between dialysis sessions. Outpatient surgical revision under local anesthesia by patch angioplasty at PTFE-vein anastomosis or extension of PTFE graft to a more proximal venous anastomotic site gives the best results.

REFERENCES

1. Kolff WJ, Berk THJ: The artificial kidney: A dialyser with a great area. *Acta Med Scand* 117:121-131, 1944.
2. Churchill DN, Taylor DW, Cook RJ, et al: Canadian Hemodialysis Morbidity Study. *Am J Kidney Dis* 19:216-234, 1995.
3. Schwab SJ, Rahmond JR, Saeed M, et al: Prevention of hemodialysis fistula thrombosis. Early detection of venous stenoses. *Kidney Int* 36:707-711, 1989.
4. Schuman E, Blayne A, Standage A, et al: Reinforced versus nonreinforced PTFE grafts for hemodialysis access. *Am J Surg* 173:407-410, 1997.
5. Cinat ME, Hopkins J, Wilson SE: A prospective evaluation of PTFE graft patency and surveillance techniques in hemodialysis access. *Ann Vasc Surg* 13:191-197, 1999.
6. Kennedy MT, Quinton H, Bubolz TA, et al: An analysis of the patency of vascular access grafts for hemodialysis using the Medicare Part B claims database. *Semin Vasc Surg* 9:262-265, 1996.
7. Hodges TC, Fillinger MF, Zwolak RM, et al: Longitudinal comparison of dialysis access methods: Risk factors for failure. *J Vasc Surg* 26:1009-1019, 1997.
8. The Vascular Access Work Group: NKF-DOQI Clinical Practice Guidelines for Vascular Access. *Am J Kidney Dis* 30:S152- S189, 1997.
9. Silva MB Jr, Hobson RW II, Papas PJ, et al: A strategy for increasing use of autogenous hemodialysis access procedures: Impact of preoperative noninvasive evaluation. *J Vasc Surg* 27:302-308, 1997.
10. Koksoy C, Kuzu A, Erden I, et al: Predictive value of color Doppler ultrasonography in detecting failure of vascular access grafts. *Br J Surg* 82:50-52, 1995.
11. Wladis AR, Mesh CL, White J, et al: Improving longevity of prosthetic dialysis grafts in patients with disadvantaged venous outflow. Presented at the 23rd Annual Meeting of the Midwestern Vascular Surgical Society, Chicago, September 25, 1999.
12. Strauch BS, O'Connell RS, Geoly KL, et al: Forecasting thrombosis of vascular access with Doppler color flow imaging. *Am J Kidney Dis* 19:554-557, 1992.
13. Sands J, Young S, Miranda C: The effect of Doppler flow screening studies and elective revisions on dialysis access failure. *Trans Am Soc Artif Intern Organs* 38:524-527, 1992.

14. Lumsden AB, MacDonald MJ, Kikeri D, et al: Cost efficacy of duplex surveillance and prophylactic angioplasty of arteriovenous ePTFE grafts. *J Vasc Surg* 26:382-390, 1997.

15. Depner TA, Rizwan S, Cheer AY, et al: High venous urea concentrations in the opposite arm: A consequence of hemodialysis-induced compartment dysequilibrium. *Trans Am Soc Artif Intern Organs* 37:141-143, 1991.

16. Shackelton CR, Taylor DC, Buckley AR, et al: Predicting failure in polytetrafluoroethylene vascular access grafts for hemodialysis: A pilot study. *Can J Surg* 30:442-444, 1987.

PART V

Pharmacologic Intervention for Peripheral Vascular Disease

CHAPTER 13

Cilostazol and the Pharmacologic Treatment of Intermittent Claudication

Jeffrey W. Kronson, MD, MSc
Fellow, Section of Vascular Surgery, Department of Cardiovascular Thoracic Surgery, Rush-Presbyterian-St. Luke's Medical Center, Chicago, Illinois

Walter J. McCarthy, MD, MS epi
Associate Professor of Surgery, Rush Medical College, Chief, Section of Vascular Surgery, Department of Cardiovascular Thoracic Surgery, Rush-Presbyterian-St. Luke's Medical Center, Chief, Division of Vascular Surgery, Cook County Hospital, Chicago, Illinois

The North American population is aging and as this cohort approaches an age greater than 65 years, it faces an ever-increasing incidence of medical diseases. Peripheral vascular disease, along with coronary artery disease, diabetes, and cancer, is one of the most prevalent medical conditions that this aging populace will encounter. Intermittent claudication is the most common manifestation of peripheral vascular disease and is on a continuum that may progress to rest pain and tissue loss. Intermittent claudication is defined as lower extremity muscular pain induced by exercise and relieved by short periods of rest. The pain is most commonly reported in the posterior aspect of the middle or lower calf. Intermittent claudication is no longer considered a benign symptom because it is a marker for coronary and cerebral atherosclerosis and remarkably occurs in 10% of persons aged 70 years or older.[1] Approximately 25% of patients with intermittent claudication will progress to severe ischemia,[2] and require an intervention to increase tissue perfusion. In fact, the cumulative lifetime amputation rate ranges from 5% to 11% for recently reported series of patients with intermittent claudication.[3] The 5-year mortality rate for this group of patients is as high as 20%, primarily because of their numerous associated comorbidities.

With the high prevalence mentioned, it is estimated that 4.7 million persons have these symptoms in the United States alone. Most do not need or want an operative intervention but are nevertheless inconvenienced by their leg pain. This situation has provided the impetus for the pharmaceutical industry to develop effective pharmacologic treatments for intermittent claudication.

The presence of physical findings suggestive of arterial occlusive disease at the first patient encounter is the most important predictor of clinical outcome in patients with intermittent claudication. This first office visit is the time to begin educating the patient regarding the risks of continued smoking and addressing the need for a diligent, graded exercise program. Other risk factors such as hypertension, diabetes, hyperlipidemia, and homocystinemia should be identified and treated. It is important to tell the patient that not all people with claudication progress to advanced ischemia. Most remain stable for years or even the duration of their lifespan with simple lifestyle modification regimens. Some younger, more active patients may require surgery or angioplasty, whereas others continue to have intermittent episodes of mild ischemia for extended periods. Some patients wish to avoid an operation or angioplasty at all costs and look for other avenues to alleviate their condition. Many of these patients would be helped with their symptoms with an effective medication.

Intermittent claudication per se is often measured by graded treadmill testing, where the patient walks a predetermined speed on a slight gradient until either completion of a certain time or the onset of symptoms. The time to onset of leg pain is referred to as the initial claudication distance (ICD), and the time to reach leg pain that forces the patient to stop walking is called the absolute claudication distance (ACD). These distances are used to compare the efficacy of different treatment groups, both pharmacologic and otherwise, in the management of this population. When initially diagnosing intermittent claudication, treadmill evaluation may not be necessary if the standard ankle-brachial index (ABI) is decreased and the patient's symptom complex is typical.

In this chapter, we first briefly examine the nonpharmacologic, nonsurgical, and noninterventional management of intermittent claudication, with emphasis on alteration in smoking and exercise. We then review a number of pharmacologic agents that have been studied to see if they decrease the symptoms of intermittent claudication. Finally, we examine in some depth the antiplatelet agent cilostazol, with a discussion of its pharmacotherapy, mechanism, and use in clinical trials.

NONOPERATIVE, NONPHARMACOLOGIC TREATMENT
CESSATION OF SMOKING

The cessation of smoking forms the foundation of the nonoperative treatment of intermittent claudication. Almost 350,000 lives are lost to tobacco every year in the United States alone, with health care costs exceeding $16 billion. Nicotine, the addictive chemical in tobacco, is responsible for symptomatology that includes arousal, relaxation, relief of hunger, and enhanced vigilance. Cessation of smoking causes withdrawal symptoms including restlessness, anxiety and sleep disturbance, weight gain, and delayed performance time.

The physiologic causes of progression of peripheral vascular disease related to smoking include the alteration of vascular endothelium, prostaglandin metabolism, platelet function, lipid metabolism, blood viscosity, and alteration in the coagulation cascade.[4] Interestingly, patients who have completely stopped smoking have been known to double their treadmill walking distances, and improved patency in arterial reconstruction, at both the aortofemoral and femoropopliteal level, has been reported.[5] Finally, amputation rates are higher for smokers who have claudication than for ex-smokers who have claudication.

Cessation of smoking occurs as patients become educated, gain a desire to improve their health, and receive encouragement from the surrounding social support structure, including family, friends, and the treating physician. The advice to stop smoking should be repeated and emphasized at every patient encounter, but one third of patients who quit do so without any kind of formal program. The advent of medical replacements for nicotine has had an impact on the withdrawal symptoms smokers face when they quit and has led to many more people attempting to quit than had previously been the case. Withdrawal symptoms can be ablated with 30% of a smoker's nicotine intake replaced. Gum, transdermal patches, an oral preparation and most recently a nicotine inhaler are all in current use.

EXERCISE

Most patients who have pain with walking intuitively believe the pain to be harmful and therefore do not continue to "walk despite the pain." In fact, it has been demonstrated that exercise is very valuable. Exercise has been shown to provide an overall improvement in both ICD and ACD of 120% to 180%.[6] It has been reported that for this effect to be seen, the patient must perform at least 30 to 60 minutes of uninterrupted walking for at least 3 days per week. Despite documented improvements in walking distance, neither an increase in ABI or calf muscle blood flow has been shown to occur.

Proposed mechanisms to explain increased walking distances after exercise include improved oxidative metabolic capacity, adaptations in walking technique, and spontaneous fluctuations in pain tolerance.[7] Finally, exercise may decrease whole blood and plasma viscosity and blood cell filterability. Overall, emphasis should be placed on the total benefits derived from an exercise program, which are obviously not limited to the patient's claudication symptoms but also include cardiopulmonary and musculoskeletal conditioning as well.

PHARMACOLOGIC TREATMENT
OVERVIEW

A number of pharmacologic agents have been studied and used clinically for patients with various degrees of intermittent claudication. Pentoxifylline, originally introduced as a vasodilator because of its effect in vitro, does not have this effect in humans but is thought to increase red cell membrane flexibility. It has been shown in vivo to increase plethysmographically measured limb and calf muscle blood flow and increase muscle Po_2.[8] Randomized trials in Europe and the United States have shown an increase in walking distance versus placebo, but the drug has been criticized because the improvements are modest. Fewer than 10% of patients have shown a 100% increase in walking distance. Side effects include dizziness and gastrointestinal symptoms. Pentoxifylline is approved for use to treat intermittent claudication by the Food and Drug Administration (FDA).

Acetylsalicylic acid (ASA) irreversibly acetylates the enzyme cyclooxygenase, blocking the synthesis of thromboxane A_2 and decreasing platelet aggregation and release. It is recommended that patients with symptoms of coronary or vascular disease use aspirin because its antiplatelet effect has been shown to decrease mortality in these groups of patients. In fact, survival in multiple groups of patients with atherosclerosis, such as those who have had a stroke or transient ischemic attack, is increased with aspirin use. Furthermore, most patients who have had arterial bypass procedures performed can benefit from its use. Recently, there are data supporting the preoperative administration of ASA to increase the patency of prosthetic reconstructions.[9] Importantly, aspirin does not alter the symptoms of intermittent claudication but rather is usually recommended to decrease ischemic events, such as stroke or myocardial infarction, thereby increasing longevity.

Ticlodipine was introduced as an inhibitor of platelet adenosine diphosphate (ADP) receptors and as an agent that reduces whole blood viscosity.[10] It has been extensively studied in Europe with inconclusive results; some reports have shown increases in walking distances and ABI, whereas others have demonstrated no benefit.[11] Side effects of the drug include a leukopenia that reverses once the drug is stopped. It currently has a limited role in the management of patients with intermittent claudication because other agents, including aspirin, have been shown to provide similar outcomes.

Other agents that are less well known deserve mention because they have been extensively studied outside North America and may hold some promise in selected groups of patients. Naftidrofuryl stimulates carbohydrates and fats to enter the tricarboxylic acid cycle, resulting in an increase in adenosine triphosphate (ATP) in ischemic areas. Results have been mixed, but the drug is widely prescribed outside the United States for patients with intermittent claudication. L-carnitine is a drug that has no known detrimental effects. It facilitates aerobic metabolism by increasing the entry of pyruvate into the citric acid cycle and the transport of cytosolic free fatty acids into the mitochondria. One mole of pyruvate produces 30 moles of ATP, which increases the muscle's work capacity.[12] Some work with this agent has shown an increase in walking distance, and consequently, the results of a US multicenter trial with the analogue L-propionyl carnitine are awaited.

Vascular surgeons occasionally encounter patients who have undergone chelation treatment with EDTA (ethylenediaminetetraaceticacid). However, no benefit has been shown with this treatment compared with placebo. One study reported no change in the pretreatment and posttreatment angiograms[13] in patients with intermittent claudication receiving EDTA. Furthermore, the cost is as much as $10,000 per treatment.

A 1994 study by Scheffler et al[14] showed a 604% increase in walking distance with prostaglandin E_1 (PGE_1), which is a prostaglandin analogue. An oral preparation is undergoing phase III multicenter testing, and the results are eagerly awaited.

CILOSTAZOL

Optimal drug treatment of intermittent claudication would include an agent that effectively increases arterial blood flow, improves oxygenation, relieves symptoms, and increases walking distance. Cilostazol has been used in Japan for more than a decade. It has been intensely studied and found to be both an inhibitor of platelet aggregation and an arterial vasodilator. It was approved for treatment of intermittent claudication by the FDA in January 1999 and is currently awaiting approval in several European countries.

Mechanism

Cilostazol selectively inhibits cyclic guanosine monophosphate (cGMP)-inhibited, cyclic adenosine monophosphate (cAMP)-selective phosphodiesterase III (PDE III), which results in an increase in intracellular cAMP, which in turn decreases intracellular calcium. This leads to inhibition of platelet aggregation and attenuated release of prothrombotic substances by both platelets and human endothelial cells (ECs). Cilostazol has been found to potentiate the anti-aggregating effect of human ECs in vitro.[15] It inhibits platelet aggregation with and without ECs, but the effect is more pronounced in the presence of ECs.[16] Given orally in a dosage of 200 mg/d, it has been found to inhibit both ADP and arachidonic acid–induced platelet aggregation in healthy volunteers.[17]

Cilostazol inhibits both primary (ADP and collagen induced) and secondary platelet aggregation, with 10 to 30 times more potency than ASA.[18] One study found cilostazol to inhibit stress-induced platelet aggregation in 6 healthy volunteers given a one-time dose of 100 mg.[19] This is of significance to vascular surgeons because stress-induced platelet aggregation has been found to be important for thrombosis at aortic bifurcations and stenotic arterial lesions. Saniabadi et al[20] found cilostazol decreased remnant lipoprotein particles of plasma chylomicrons and very low density lipoproteins, which are also responsible for the platelet aggregation that leads to atherosclerosis.

In a multicenter, randomized, double-blind trial, patients received 100 mg of cilostazol orally twice a day. Higher levels of apolipoprotein A and high-density lipoprotein cholesterol were found in these patients compared with controls, as well as lower triglyceride levels, although the clinical significance of these findings has not been formally subjected to scientific scrutiny.[21] Cilostazol has also been found to inhibit monocyte chemoattractant protein-1 (MCP-1), through the increased levels of cAMP.[22] MCP-1 stimulation by tumor necrosis factor was inhibited as well. These findings suggest that cilostazol may have a role to play in the injury-response theory of atherogenesis. Nomura et al[23] found that cilostazol decreased levels of platelet-derived microparticles

(PMP), as well as levels of activated platelets and soluble adhesion molecules.[23] The sum of these findings was that the drug would be useful in both PMP-dependent and PMP-independent vascular damage in type 2 diabetes mellitus.

Cilostazol also has an arterial vasodilatory effect. An increase in cAMP has been shown in isolated rabbit aortic strips.[24] The release of calcium is blocked, and therefore, little or no smooth muscle contraction occurs. This effect is found to be nonhomogeneous; femoral arteries are affected more than vertebral and superior mesenteric arteries, and renal arteries are not affected at all.

Pharmacokinetics

Cilostazol is a 2-oxoquinolone with a half-life of 18 to 25.5 hours. Its time to maximum blood level is 0.5 to 4 hours. These kinetics are not affected by age or gender.[25] Ninety-five percent of the drug is protein bound in plasma, primarily to albumin. Seventy-one percent is excreted in urine, through 2 active metabolites: (1) monohydroxycilostazol, which is 3 times less potent than the parent compound; and (2) dehydrocilostazol, which is 3 times more potent.

The clearance of dehydrocilostazol can be delayed with concomitant administration of omeprazole or erythromycin, because dehydrocilostazol is metabolized through a common cytochrome p450 pathway, using CYP3A4.[26] However, there is no drug interaction with either ASA or warfarin and no effect on prothrombin time, partial thromboplastin time, or bleeding time. The clearance of the drug is increased with severe renal disease (spillage) and is decreased with hepatic disease (suboptimal metabolism).

Cilostazol is contraindicated in congestive heart failure because PDE III inhibitors may increase mortality through the production of lethal dysrhythmias, caused by high levels of cAMP.

Clinical Trials

A number of small and large clinical studies have been performed both in the United States and in Japan to test the hypothesis that cilostazol will positively affect the natural history of intermittent claudication, by inhibiting atherosclerosis through inhibition of platelet function and increasing blood flow by arterial vasodilation.

Kamiya and Sakaguchi[27] found that in patients with chronic arterial occlusion, 150 mg of cilostazol given orally twice a day was able to increase mean blood flow, as measured by the venous occlusion method, by 16.2%. They postulated that the increase in blood flow in patients with type 2 diabetes mellitus might prevent nerve tissue ischemia and neuropathy. In another study, Uchikawa et al[28] found increases in skin temperature with daily oral doses of 200 to 300 mg, suggesting a peripheral vasodilatory effect.

Cilostazol has been studied extensively in coronary artery disease as well. One study found that patients given 200 mg of cilostazol orally per day before undergoing coronary atherectomy had larger postatherectomy diameters when followed up to 6 months compared with controls and those given ASA.[29] In this series, the restenosis rate was 0% (n = 21) for those patients receiving cilostazol and 26% (n = 20) for those taking ASA. However, Park et al[30] found no difference in 30-day major cardiac events or adverse drug effects in patients undergoing coronary stenting and receiving ASA plus either cilostazol or ticlodipine.[30]

Six large multicenter trials have been undertaken in the United States to test the efficacy of cilostazol to modify the symptoms of intermittent claudication (Table 1).

Beebe et al[31] studied 516 patients who were entered in a randomized, double-blinded study. They were given cilostazol, either 50 or 100 mg/d orally, or placebo. The authors found a dose-dependent increase in ICD (59%) and ACD (51%) versus placebo. The results were confirmed by 3 separate subscales of the short-form health survey, including one measuring physical functioning. Of the 516 patients, 31% taking the drug reported headache, 27% diarrhea, and 8% palpitations.

Dawson et al[32] described 81 patients who were entered in a prospective, randomized, double-blinded study. All had moderate intermittent claudication. Fifty-two patients received cilostazol, 100 mg orally twice a day, and 25 received placebo. Effects were seen after 12 weeks with a 58% increase in ICD and a 63% increase in ACD over baseline. Forty-four percent had gastrointestinal side effects (15% for placebo), and 20% reported headache (15% for placebo).

Strandness et al[33] studied 394 patients for 24 weeks. They received cilostazol, either 50 or 100 mg/d orally, or placebo. An increase in ICD (22%) and ACD (21%) versus placebo was observed.

Money et al,[34] in a randomized, double-blinded, placebo-controlled trial, followed up 239 patients in 17 centers. The patients received cilostazol, 100 mg/d orally, or placebo. The authors found an increased time to initial onset of symptoms and a 47% increase in maximum walking distance over baseline. Up to 55% of study group patients reported feeling better after starting the drug. Notably, they also found an increase in the baseline ABI of 9.0%

TABLE 1.
Recent US Multicenter Trials Evaluating Cilostazol

Author	Year	Patients (N)	Dosage (mg)	Results
Beebe et al[31]	1997	516	50/100 qd	ICD ^ 59%, ACD ^ 51% vs placebo
Dawson et al[32]	1998	81	100 bid	ICD ^ 58%, ACD ^ 63% vs baseline
Strandness et al[33]	1998	394	50/100 qd	ICD ^ 22%, ACD ^ 21% vs placebo
Money et al[34]	1998	239	100 bid	ACD ^ 47% vs baseline, ABI ^ 9.0% vs 1.5% for placebo
Elam et al[35]	1998	189	100 bid	ACD ^ 36% vs 24% for placebo, ABI ^ 11% vs baseline
Dawson et al[36]	1998	698	100 bid vs 400 tid pentoxifylline	ICD ^ 98%, ACD ^ 54% vs baseline ACD ^ 30% for pentoxifylline

Abbreviations: ICD, Initial claudication distance; *ACD,* absolute claudication distance; *ABI,* ankle-brachial index; *qd,* every day; *bid,* twice a day; *tid,* 3 times a day.

versus 1.5% with placebo. Thirty percent of patients taking the drug reported headache, 29% abnormal stools, and 13% dizziness.

Elam et al,[35] in a randomized, double-blinded study lasting 12 weeks, evaluated 189 patients with intermittent claudication. They also received cilostazol, 100 mg/d orally. The authors reported an increase in ACD of 35.5% versus 24.3% with placebo. Furthermore, those members of the study group were found to have an 11.1% increase in their baseline ABI compared with no increase in those patients in the placebo group.

Dawson et al[36] enrolled 698 patients with claudication in a randomized, double-blinded, placebo-controlled trial. They received either cilostazol, 100 mg orally twice a day, or pentoxifylline, 400 mg orally 3 times a day. Those in the cilostazol group were found to have increases in pain-free walking distance (98% over baseline, $P < .05$) and ACD (54% over baseline compared with 30% for pentoxifylline and 34% for placebo, $P < .05$). Furthermore, withdrawal of cilostazol, not pentoxifylline, worsened walking distance.

CONCLUSIONS AND FUTURE DIRECTIONS

Intermittent claudication is a disease facing an increasing percentage of our population as it ages and an ever larger cohort passes 65 years. With the evolution of less invasive therapies for a variety of disease processes and the advancement of our understanding of molecular biology and pharmacotherapeutics, it is not surprising that alternative therapies for peripheral vascular disease other than surgery or angioplasty arise. Cessation of smoking, a graded exercise program, and an inexpensive antiplatelet agent such as ASA remain the mainstays of treatment. However, a number of new drug agents are becoming available in the armamentarium of the vascular physician or surgeon. Of these, cilostazol, a potent PDE III inhibitor, should be considered for many patients because it has been conclusively and repetitively shown to inhibit platelet aggregation and vasodilate arteries in vitro and has been demonstrated, through a number of well-controlled clinical trials, to prolong both ICD and ACD. Furthermore, it is reasonably well tolerated, with mild gastrointestinal side effects and headache being the most commonly reported adverse events. In a recently reported head-to-head clinical trial, cilostazol outperformed pentoxifylline, the only other drug currently approved for treatment of intermittent claudication in the United States. Final results from additional trials of such agents as PGE_1 and L-carnitine are anticipated in the near future.

REFERENCES

1. Peabody CN, Kannel WB, McNamara PM: Intermittent claudication: Surgical significance. *Arch Surg* 109:639-697, 1974.
2. Rosenbloom MS, Flanigan DP, Schuler JJ, et al: Risk factors affecting the history of intermittent claudication. *Arch Surg* 123:867-870, 1998.
3. Nehler MR, Taylor LM, Moneta GL, et al: Natural history, nonoperative treatment, and functional assessment in chronic lower extremity ischemia, in Moore WS (ed): *Vascular Surgery: A Comprehensive Review* 5th ed. Philadelphia, WB Saunders Co, 1998, p 251.
4. Krupski WC, Rapp JH: Smoking and atherosclerosis. *Perspect Vasc Surg* 1:103-134, 1989.
5. Provan JL, Sojka SG, Murnaghan JJ, et al: The effect of cigarette smoking on the long term success rate of aortofemoral and femoropopliteal reconstructions. *Surg Gynecol Obstet* 165:49-52, 1987.
6. Gardner AW, Poehlman ET: Exercise rehabilitation programs for clau-

dication pain: A meta-analysis. *JAMA* 274:975-980, 1995.

7. Dahlof AG, Bjorntorp P, Holm J, et al: Metabolic activity of skeletal muscles in patients with peripheral arterial insufficiency. *Eur J Clin Invest* 4:9-15, 1974.

8. Ehrly AM: Effects of orally administered pentoxifylline on muscular oxygen pressure in patients with intermittent claudication. *IRCS Med Sci* 10:401-402, 1982.

9. Clagett GP, Genton E, Salzman EW: Antithrombotic therapy in peripheral vascular disease. *Chest* 95:1286-1298, 1989.

10. Panak E, Maffrand JP, Picard-Fraire C, et al: Ticlodipine: A promise for the prevention and treatment of thrombosis and its complications. *Haemostasis* 13:1S-52S, 1983.

11. Fagher B, for the STIMS Group: Long-term effects of ticlodipine on lower limb blood flow, ankle/brachial index and symptoms in peripheral arteriosclerosis: A double-blind study. *Angiology* 45:777-788, 1994.

12. Goa KL, Brogden RN: L-carnitine: A preliminary review of its pharmacokinetics, and its therapeutic use in ischemic heart disease and primary and secondary carnitine deficiencies in relationship to its role in fatty acid metabolism. *Drugs* 34:1-24, 1987.

13. Guldager B, Jelnes R, Jorgensen SJ, et al: EDTA treatment of intermittent claudication: A double-blind, placebo-controlled study. *J Intern Med* 231:261-267, 1992.

14. Scheffler P, de la Hamette D, Gross J, et al: Intensive vascular training in stage IIb of peripheral arterial occlusive disease. The additive effects of Prostaglandin E1, or intravenous pentoxifylline during training. *Circulation* 90(2):818-822, 1994.

15. Tajima M, Maruyama S, Sato S: The role of endothelial cells in the antithrombotic effect of cilostazol. (abstract). *Jpn J Pharmacol* 55 Suppl 1:145, 1991.

16. Igawa T, Tani T, Chijiwa T, et al: Potentiation of anti-platelet aggregating activity of cilostazol with vascular endothelial cells. *Thromb Res* 57:617-623, 1990.

17. Shimodaira H, Shibuya H, Uchida K, et al: Clinical study of some platelet antiaggregation agents on healthy volunteers. *Rinsho Yakuri* 21:605-612, 1990.

18. Comp PC: Treatment of intermittent claudication in peripheral vascular disease: Recent clinical experience with cilostazol. *Today's Therapeutic Trends* 17:99-112, 1999.

19. Minami N, Suzuki Y, Yamamoto M, et al: Inhibition of shear stress-induced platelet aggregation by cilostazol, a specific inhibitor of cGMP-inhibited phosphodiesterase, *in vitro* and *ex vivo*. *Life Sci* 61:383-389, 1997.

20. Saniabadi AR, Takeich S, Yukawa N, et al: Apo E4/3-rich remnant lipoproteins and platelet aggregation: A case report. *Thromb Haemost* 79:878-879, 1998.

21. Elam MB, Heckman J, Crouse JR, et al: Effect of the novel antiplatelet

agent cilostazol on plasma lipoproteins in patients with intermittent claudication. *Arterioscler Thromb Vasc Biol* 18:1942-1947, 1998.

22. Nishio Y, Kashiwagi A, Takahara N, et al: Cilostazol, a cAMP phosphodiesterase inhibitor, attenuates the production of monocyte chemoattractant protein-1 in response to tumor necrosis factor-alpha in vascular endothelial cells. *Horm Metab Res* 29:491-495, 1997.

23. Nomura S, Shouza A, Omoto S, et al: Effect of cilostazol on soluble molecules and platelet-derived microparticles in patients with diabetes. *Thromb Haemost* 80:388-392, 1998.

24. Tanaka T, Ishikawa T, Hagiwara M, et al: Effects of cilostazol, a selective cAMP phosphodiesterase inhibitor on the contraction of vascular smooth muscle. *Pharmacology* 36:313-320, 1988.

25. Suri A, Forbes WP, Bramer SL: Pharmacokinetics of multiple-dose oral cilostazol in middle-age and elderly men and women. *J Clin Pharmacol* 38:144-150, 1998.

26. Suri A, Forbes WP, Bramer SL: The effects of CYP3A4 inhibition by erythromycin on the metabolism of cilostazol. *Pharm Res* 14:562S, 1997.

27. Kamiya T, Sakaguchi S: Hemodynamic effects of the antithrombotic drug cilostazol in chronic arterial occlusion in the extremities. *Arzneimittelforschung* 35:1201-1203, 1985.

28. Uchikawa T, Murakami T, Furukawa H: Effects of the anti-platelet agent cilostazol on peripheral vascular disease in patients with diabetes mellitus. *Arzneimittelforschung* 42:322-324, 1992.

29. Tsuchikane E, Katoh O, Sumitsuji S, et al: Impact of cilostazol on intimal proliferation after directional coronary atherectomy. *Am Heart J* 135:495-502, 1998.

30. Park SW, Lee CW, Kim HS, et al: Comparison of cilostazol versus ticlodipine after stent implantation. *Am J Cardiol* 84:511-514, 1999.

31. Beebe HG, Dawson DL, Cutler BS, et al: Cilostazol, a new treatment for intermittent claudication: Results of a randomized, multicenter trial. *Circulation* 96:I-12S, 1997.

32. Dawson DL, Cutler BS, Meissner MH, et al: Cilostazol has beneficial effects in treatment of intermittent claudication. Results from a multicenter, randomized, prospective, double-blind trial. *Circulation* 98:678-686, 1998.

33. Strandness DE, Dalman R, Panian S, et al: Two doses of cilostazol versus placebo in the treatment of claudication: Results of a randomized, multicenter trial. *Circulation* 98:I-12, 1998.

34. Money SR, Herd JA, Isaacsohn JL, et al: Effect of cilostazol on walking distances in patients with intermittent claudication caused by peripheral vascular disease. *J Vasc Surg* 27:267-275, 1998.

35. Elam MB, Heckman J, Crouse JR, et al: Effect of the novel antiplatelet agent cilostazol on plasma lipoproteins in patients with intermittent claudication. *Arterioscler Thromb Vasc Biol* 18:1942-1947, 1998.

36. Dawson DL, Beebe HG, Davidson M, et al: Cilostazol or pentoxifylline for claudication? *Circulation* 98:I-12, 1998.

CHAPTER 14

Statin Therapy in Atherosclerosis

Joshua A. Beckman, MD
Instructor of Medicine, Harvard University Medical School; Associate
Attending Vascular Medicine Section, Cardiovascular Division,
Department of Medicine, Brigham and Women's Hospital, Boston

The complications of atherosclerosis, including heart attack, stroke, and amputation, are the leading causes of morbidity and mortality in the United States. Among physicians, vascular surgeons have unique access to patients with peripheral atherosclerosis. This access gives them an opportunity to affect the short- and long-term consequences of atherosclerosis. Because symptomatic atherosclerosis in one vascular bed increases the chance of subclinical atherosclerosis in another, the initiation of proper medical therapy reduces the likelihood of future clinical events, even in asymptomatic areas. Standard medical therapy for patients with atherosclerotic vascular disease includes risk-factor modification. Among the important interventions made by physicians, treating hypercholesterolemia reaps important and proved benefits. One class of cholesterol-lowering medications, the 3-hydroxyl-3-methyl-glutaryl coenzyme A (HMG-CoA) reductase inhibitors, better known as statins, has been shown in many clinical settings to decrease the morbidity and mortality of patients with atherosclerosis.

This review will discuss the mechanism of action of statins, review the link between elevated levels of total or low-density lipoprotein (LDL) cholesterol and atherosclerosis in the various vascular beds, examine the clinical data supporting statin use, survey the relationship between peripheral and coronary atherosclerosis, and discuss nationally accepted guidelines for statin use.

MECHANISM OF ACTION OF STATINS

The rate-limiting enzyme for cholesterol synthesis in the liver is HMG-CoA reductase. Administration of an HMG-CoA reductase

inhibitor reduces the hepatic production and content of cholesterol and increases the expression of the LDL receptors. These
receptors are responsible for LDL uptake through endocytosis. The
result is normal cellular cholesterol content and lower plasma concentration.[1] In addition to the plasma LDL-lowering effect, statins
modestly reduce the plasma triglyceride level and increase high-
density lipoprotein (HDL) concentrations.

The statins vary in absorption rate, mechanism of excretion, sol-
ubility, and extent of LDL lowering, although no comparative data
exist to suggest that one agent is more protective against cardiovascular events than another (Table 1). The most common side
effects are myositis and transient elevations in serum hepatic
transaminases. Both of these occur infrequently and tend to
resolve with the cessation of statin use. Coadministration of fibric-
acid derivatives, macrolide antibiotics, or cyclosporine increases
the risk of myositis.

Of interest, statins recently have been shown to exert other
pharmacological effects that may reduce the risk of vascular morbidity and mortality. For example, HMG-CoA reductase inhibitors
increase the production of endothelial nitric oxide synthase in
vitro, independent of their effects on cholesterol.[2] Diminished
bioavailability of endothelium-derived nitric oxide is an early
manifestation of atherosclerosis, and increases in nitric oxide synthase may improve endothelial function and retard the progression
of atherosclerosis. Indeed, HMG-CoA reductase inhibitors, acting
through endothelial nitric oxide synthase, have afforded stroke
protection in rats.[3] Research concerning benefits other than cholesterol lowering is ongoing.

TABLE 1.

Characteristics of FDA-approved Statins

Agent	Dose Range (mg/day)	Renal Excretion (%)	Cholesterol Reduction	
			Total (%)	LDL (%)
Atorvastatin calcium	10 to 80	2	27 to 42	27 to 55
Cerivastatin sodium	0.2 to 0.3	24	22 to 27	27 to 34
Fluvastatin sodium	20 to 80	6	22 to 27	27 to 34
Lovastatin	20 to 80	30	22 to 32	27 to 41
Pravastatin sodium	10 to 40	60	22 to 27	27 to 24
Simvastatin	5 to 80	13	22 to 37	27 to 48

Abbreviations: LDL, low-density lipoprotein.

HYPERCHOLESTEROLEMIA AND ATHEROSCLEROSIS
CORONARY ARTERY DISEASE

The Framingham Heart Study established the link between total cholesterol and the development of coronary artery disease.[4] Confirming this relationship, the Multiple Risk Factor Intervention Trial (MRFIT) screened and followed more than 350,000 men for at least 6 years and showed a curvilinear relationship between total cholesterol and coronary artery disease mortality. The risk increased directly with levels above 200 mg/dL and more dramatically at levels above 280 mg/dL.[5] This association has been extended to women, young men, and the elderly and correlated in patients with established coronary artery disease.

Based on the epidemiological association between elevated serum cholesterol and coronary artery disease, trials were conducted to examine whether reducing cholesterol levels would reduce the risks of heart attack and death. Primary-prevention studies revealed that lowering the total or LDL cholesterol level reduced the incidence of nonfatal myocardial infarction, but a meta-analysis of 4 nonstatin trials showed no reduction in fatal myocardial infarction.[6] Secondary-prevention trials were more successful. The Stockholm Ischaemic Heart Disease Secondary Prevention Study, which tested clofibrate and nicotinic acid, showed that a 13% decrease in serum cholesterol resulted in a 36% reduction in cardiovascular mortality.[7] Furthermore, in the Program On the Surgical Control of Hyperlipidemia (POSCH), patients were randomly assigned to partial ileal bypass or dietary advice. Patients who underwent bypass had a 23% lower total cholesterol level and 35% fewer total cardiac events.[8] These trials confirmed the causative link between increased serum levels of total and LDL cholesterol and symptomatic coronary artery disease.

PERIPHERAL ARTERIAL DISEASE

The relationship between total and LDL cholesterol levels and lower-extremity atherosclerosis has been shown in large epidemiological trials, such as the Framingham study[9] and the Edinburgh artery study.[10] Elevated total cholesterol and LDL levels increase the risk of lower-extremity atherosclerosis, although the increase is less than that associated with cigarette smoking and diabetes mellitus.[11] Each 10-mg/dL increase in total serum cholesterol increases the risk ratio by 1.1.[12] No prospective trial has shown an improvement in the progression of lower-extremity atherosclerosis; however, the POSCH trial showed a decrease in new-onset claudication with cholesterol lowering.[8]

Serum cholesterol levels do not have a predictable effect on the risk of stroke. In fact, lower cholesterol levels may actually increase the risk of hemorrhagic stroke.[13] Furthermore, a meta-analysis of lipid-lowering trials using nonstatin cholesterol-lowering drugs or diet showed a decrease in nonfatal stroke and an increase in fatal stroke.[14]

STATIN CLINICAL TRIALS

In determining the benefits of statins in patients with atherosclerosis, one must consider that large clinical trials have investigated the benefits of statin-related cholesterol lowering only in relation to coronary artery disease events. Information about the effects of statins on symptomatic cerebrovascular and peripheral arterial disease can be gleaned only from secondary endpoints, retrospective determinations, and meta-analyses of the aforementioned studies. Therefore, the cardiovascular benefit will be discussed first, followed by the outcomes in cerebrovascular and peripheral vascular disease.

BENEFITS IN CORONARY ARTERY DISEASE

Large clinical trials have established the benefits of statins in several important clinical settings: primary prevention, secondary prevention, and secondary prevention after surgical revascularization (Table 2).[15-24]

Primary Prevention

The West Of Scotland Coronary Prevention Study (WOSCOPS) was the first landmark trial to show the relationship between total and LDL cholesterol reduction and the primary prevention of myocardial infarction, death from coronary artery disease, and all-cause mortality.[15] Nearly 6600 men with no previous myocardial infarction and an average total cholesterol of 272 mg/dL and LDL cholesterol of 192 mg/dL were randomized to receive pravastatin or matching placebo each day. The patients were followed up for 4.9 years. Patients treated with pravastatin reduced their total cholesterol level by an average of 20%, and LDL cholesterol by 26%. Treated patients showed a 31% decrease in nonfatal myocardial infarction or death from coronary artery disease and a 37% decrease in percutaneous or surgical revascularization. There was a borderline significant ($P = .051$) improvement in all-cause mortality.

More recently, the same level of benefit in primary prevention has been shown in patients with an average cholesterol level. The Air Force/Texas Coronary Atherosclerosis Prevention Study (AFCAPS/TexCAPS) enrolled 5608 middle-aged men and 997 postmenopausal women who had a total cholesterol level of 221

TABLE 2.
Prospective, Large Statin Trials

Clinical Trial	Study Attributes	Duration (y)	LDL (%)	CAD Mortality (%)	CABG or PTCA (%)	Stroke (%)
				Reduction		
WOSCOPS[15]	EC, A, P	4.9	26	28	37	11 (NS)
AFCAPS/ TexCAPS[16]	NC, A, L	5.2	25	36	33	NA
4S[17,18,23]	EC, CAD, S	5	35	42	37	30
CARE[19,21,24]	NC, CAD, P	5	28	19	27	31
LIPID[20]	NC, CAD, P	6.1	25	24	22*	19
Post-CABG[22]	NC, CABG, L	4-5	40	NA	29	NA

*CABG alone. *Abbreviations: A,* asymptomatic; *AC,* average cholesterol; *CABG,* coronary artery bypass graft; *CAD,* coronary artery disease; *EC,* elevated cholesterol; *L,* lovastatin; *NA,* not available; *AC,* average cholesterol; *NS,* not significant; *P,* pravastatin; *S,* simvastatin.

mg/dL and an LDL cholesterol level of 150 mg/dL and treated them with lovastatin or matching placebo.[16] With lovastatin therapy, total and LDL cholesterol levels declined by 18% and 25%, respectively, and the primary end point of fatal or nonfatal myocardial infarction, unstable angina, or sudden death decreased by 37%. There also was a significant decrease in the frequency of coronary artery revascularization.

Secondary Prevention
The first major study to evaluate the benefit of statins in prevention of coronary events in patients with symptomatic coronary disease was the Scandinavian Simvastatin Survival Study (4S).[17] This trial examined the benefit of cholesterol lowering in 4444 patients with increased cholesterol levels and angina pectoris or previous myocardial infarction. Simvastatin reduced total and LDL cholesterol levels by 25% and 35%, respectively. Over the 5 years of follow-up, there was a 42% reduction in coronary-related death and a 30% reduction in all-cause mortality. This benefit extended to subgroups stratified by sex, smoking status, age, and hypertension.[18] Of interest, patients with diabetes mellitus showed a much greater improvement with treatment than did the other subgroups, which confirms the requirement for increased vigilance in this group.[17]

The Cholesterol and Recurrent Events (CARE) trial investigators examined the benefit of pravastatin sodium related cholesterol lowering in 4159 patients with myocardial infarction and average total and LDL cholesterol levels of 209 and 139 mg/dL, respectively.[19] During the 5-year follow-up, there was a 24% reduction in death from coronary disease or nonfatal MI and a 27% reduction in percutaneous or surgical revascularization. The Long-term Intervention with Pravastatin in Ischemic Disease (LIPID) trial similarly confirmed the benefits of statin-related cholesterol lowering in 9014 patients who had an average cholesterol level.[20]

Benefits After Revascularization

The treatment benefit in patients with symptomatic coronary disease has been extended to patients who have undergone surgical revascularization (ie, those with the most severe atherosclerosis). The Post-Coronary Artery Bypass Graft (Post-CABG) trial enrolled 1351 subjects 1 to 11 years after surgery, thus avoiding the early graft closure usually unrelated to occlusive lesion development.[22] Patients were treated with lovastatin to achieve an LDL level below 85 mg/dL or below 140 mg/dL. Angiography performed 4 to 5 years after enrollment showed fewer occlusions, new lesions, or grafts with lesion progression in the patients with a lower LDL level, irrespective of graft age. Supporting this conclusion, the CARE investigators examined their population retrospectively and noted that cholesterol lowering conferred the same level of benefit in patients who had undergone surgical or percutaneous revascularization.[21]

BENEFITS IN CEREBROVASCULAR DISEASE

There are no prospective data to evaluate the benefits of statin therapy specifically for stroke prevention. Stroke has been evaluated as a secondary endpoint in 2 of the postinfarction trials: 4S[23] and CARE.[24] Statin therapy reduced the rate of stroke or transient ischemic attack by 30% and 27%, respectively, in these patients with elevated and average cholesterol levels.[23, 24] Meta-analyses of both primary- and secondary-prevention trials of statins in cardiovascular disease also corroborate a significant reduction in and class effect for stroke, although the primary-prevention trials alone did not reach statistical significance.[25] The 4S investigators also prospectively analyzed the frequency of subclinical disease. Statin-treated patients showed a 48% reduction in the risk of carotid bruits.[23]

BENEFITS IN LOWER-EXTREMITY ARTERIAL DISEASE

The data supporting statin use to prevent the progression of lower-extremity arterial disease are less extensive than those available for cerebrovascular disease. The only trial to evaluate the benefits of statin therapy on lower-extremity arterial disease is the 4S trial. Treated patients showed a 38% risk reduction for new intermittent claudication, but the frequency of new femoral-artery bruits did not differ.[23]

PERIPHERAL ATHEROSCLEROSIS AND CORONARY ARTERY DISEASE

Statins have undergone extensive testing, and their benefits in the primary and secondary prevention of coronary events are well-established. In patients with symptomatic coronary atherosclerosis, outcomes in the cerebrovascular circulation and lower extremities are improved with statin monotherapy. The justification for statin therapy in patients with cerebrovascular or lower-extremity atherosclerosis derives from their increased likelihood of future coronary atherosclerosis.

Both subclinical and symptomatic lower-extremity or carotid arteriosclerosis increase the risk of coronary artery disease, myocardial infarction, or death. Increasing carotid intima thickness, a measure of subclinical atherosclerosis, is associated with increased cardiovascular morbidity and mortality.[26] In 295 consecutive patients with cerebrovascular disease who underwent angiography, 60% had at least 1 diseased coronary artery.[27] During a 20-year follow-up after carotid endarterectomy, the risk of death from coronary artery disease was higher among these patients than among those without cerebrovascular disease. In fact, the risk of death from ischemic coronary disease was 3 times greater than that from cerebrovascular disease, despite the fact that these patients initially came to medical attention for symptomatic carotid disease.[28]

The relationship between lower-extremity atherosclerosis and coronary artery disease also is clear. Hertzer and colleagues performed coronary angiography in 1000 consecutive patients with surgical cerebrovascular disease, lower-extremity atherosclerotic disease, and abdominal aortic aneurysm. Of the patients with lower-extremity atherosclerosis, nearly 70% also had significant coronary artery disease.[29] In fact, the severity of lower-extremity arteriosclerosis has correlated strongly with the likelihood of myocardial infarction or death.[30] As the ankle-brachial index decreases, the probability of myocardial infarction or death increases proportionally.[31] The strong relationship between coronary artery disease and the symptomatic, atherosclerotic peripheral vascular beds typically encountered by vascular surgeons forms the basis for the therapeutic recommendations below.

THERAPEUTIC RECOMMENDATIONS

Based on prospective data from trials, any patient at high risk for or with evidence of coronary artery disease who has an increased

TABLE 3.
National Cholesterol Education Program Recommendations[32]

LDL Cholesterol (mg/dL)	Number of Risk Factors*	Physician Intervention
Less than 130		Advice on diet and exercise Recheck LDL within 5 years
130 to 159	Fewer than 2	Advice on diet and exercise Recheck LDL annually
130 to 159+	Any vascular disease	Advice on diet and exercise Statin therapy
160 to 190	Two or more risk factors or any vascualr disease	Advice on diet and exercise Statin therapy
More than 190		Advice on diet and exercise Statin therapy

*Risk factors include diabetes mellitus, cigarette smoking, hypertension, positive family history, and hypercholesterolemia. *Abbreviations: LDL,* low-density lipoprotein.

or average serum LDL cholesterol level should be treated with a statin. In patients with lower-extremity or cerebrovascular atherosclerosis, the treatment mandate exists not on the basis of secondary endpoints and retrospective evaluations of studies, but on the increased risks of myocardial infarction and death predicted by atherosclerosis in any vascular bed. Treatment guidelines have been codified by the National Cholesterol Education Program (Table 3).[32] All patients with atherosclerosis and an LDL cholesterol level above 130 mg/dL should be started on a statin. Patients with no evidence of atherosclerosis, but who have 2 or more coronary risk factors (positive family history, cigarette smoking, hypertension, diabetes, or increased cholesterol) and an LDL cholesterol level above 160 mg/dL also should receive a statin. The goal of therapy is to achieve an LDL level of less than 100 mg/dL. Although statins vary in their ability to reduce total and LDL cholesterol levels, no trial has shown the superiority of one statin over another in the prevention of clinical events. The HMG-CoA reductase inhibitors have revolutionized the treatment of hypercholesterolemia and can now be considered mandatory therapy for any patient with atherosclerosis.

REFERENCES

1. Brown MS, Goldstein JL: Multivalent feedback regulation of HMG CoA reductase, a control mechanism coordinating isoprenoid synthesis and cell growth. *J Lipid Res* 21:505517, 1980.

2. Laufs U, Liao JK: Post-transcriptional regulation of endothelial nitric oxide synthase mRNA stability by rho GTPase. *J Biol Chem* 273:24266-24271, 1998.

3. Endres M, Laufs U, Huang Z, et al: Stroke protection by 3-hydroxy-3-methylglutaryl (HMG)-CoA reductase inhibitors by endothelial nitric oxide synthase. *Proc Natl Acad Sci U S A* 95:8880-8885, 1998.

4. Kannel WB, Castelli WP, Gordon T, et al: Serum cholesterol, lipoproteins, and the risk of coronary heart disease. *Ann Intern Med* 74:1-12, 1971.

5. Stamler J, Wentworth D, Neaton JD: Is relationship between serum cholesterol and risk of premature death from coronary heart disease continuous and graded? Findings in 356,222 primary screenees of the Multiple Risk Factor Intervention Trial (MRFIT). *JAMA* 256:2823-2828, 1986.

6. Rossouw JE: The effects of lowering serum cholesterol on coronary heart disease risk. *Med Clin North Am* 78:181-195, 1994.

7. Carlson LA, Rosenhamer G: Reduction of mortality in the Stockholm Ischaemic Heart Disease Secondary Prevention Study by combined treatment with clofibrate and nicotinic acid. *Acta Med Scand* 223:405-418, 1998.

8. Buchwald H, Varco RL, Matts JP, et al: Effect of partial ileal bypass surgery on mortality and morbidity from coronary heart disease in patients with hypercholesterolemia. Report of the Program On the Surgical Control of the Hyperlipidemias (POSCH). *N Engl J Med* 323:946-955, 1990.

9. Murabito JM, D'Agostino RB, Silbershatz H, et al: Intermittent claudication: a risk profile from the Framingham Heart Study. *Circulation* 96:44-49, 1997.

10. Fowkes FG, Housley E, Riemersma RA, et al: Smoking, lipids, glucose intolerance, and blood pressure as risk factors for peripheral atherosclerosis compared with ischemic heart disease in the Edinburgh Artery Study. *Am J Epidemiol* 135:331-340, 1992.

11. Hiatt WR, Hoag S, Hamman RF: Effect of diagnostic criteria on the prevalence of peripheral arterial disease. The San Luis Valley Diabetes Study. *Circulation* 91:1472-1479, 1995.

12. Newman AB, Siscovick DS, Manolio TA, et al: Ankle-arm index as a marker of atherosclerosis in the Cardiovascular Health Study. Cardiovascular Heart Study (CHS) Collaborative Research Group. *Circulation* 88:837-845, 1993.

13. Iso H, Jacobs DRJ, Wentworth D, et al: Serum cholesterol levels and six-year mortality from stroke in 350,977 men screened for the Multiple Risk Factor Intervention Trial. *N Engl J Med* 320:904-910, 1989.

14. Atkins D, Psaty BM, Koepsell TD, et al: Cholesterol reduction and the risk for stroke in men: a meta-analysis of randomized, controlled trials. *Ann Intern Med* 119:136-145, 1993.

15. Shepherd J, Cobbe SM, Ford I, et al: Prevention of coronary heart dis-

ease with pravastatin in men with hypercholesterolemia. West Of Scotland Coronary Prevention Study Group. *N Engl J Med* 333:1301-1307, 1995.

16. Downs JR, Clearfield M, Weis S, et al: Primary prevention of acute coronary events with lovastatin in men and women with average cholesterol levels: results of AFCAPS/TexCAPS. Air Force/Texas Coronary Atherosclerosis Prevention Study. *JAMA* 279:1615-1622, 1998.

17. Randomised trial of cholesterol lowering in 4444 patients with coronary heart disease: the Scandinavian Simvastatin Survival Study (4S). *Lancet* 344:1383-1389, 1994.

18. Kjekshus J, Pedersen TR: Reducing the risk of coronary events: evidence from the Scandinavian Simvastatin Survival Study (4S). *Am J Cardiol* 76:64C-68C, 1995.

19. Sacks FM, Pfeffer MA, Moye LA, et al: The effect of pravastatin on coronary events after myocardial infarction in patients with average cholesterol levels. Cholesterol And Recurrent Events Trial investigators. *N Engl J Med* 335:1001-1009, 1996.

20. The Long-Term Intervention with Pravastatin in Ischaemic Disease (LIPID) Study Group: Prevention of cardiovascular events and death with pravastatin in patients with coronary heart disease and a broad range of initial cholesterol levels. *N Engl J Med* 339:1349-1357, 1998.

21. Flaker GC, Warnica JW, Sacks FM, et al: Pravastatin prevents clinical events in revascularized patients with average cholesterol concentrations. Cholesterol And Recurrent Events (CARE) Investigators. *J Am Coll Cardiol* 34:106-112, 1999.

22. The Post Coronary Artery Bypass Graft Trial Investigators. The effect of aggressive lowering of low-density lipoprotein cholesterol levels and low-dose anticoagulation on obstructive changes in saphenous-vein coronary-artery bypass grafts. *N Engl J Med* 336:153-162, 1997. Erratum published *N Engl J Med* 337:1859, 1997.

23. Pedersen TR, Kjekshus J, Pyorala K, et al: Effect of simvastatin on ischemic signs and symptoms in the Scandinavian Simvastatin Survival study (4S). *Am J Cardiol* 81:333-335, 1998.

24. Plehn JF, Davis BR, Sacks FM, et al: Reduction of stroke incidence after myocardial infarction with pravastatin: the Cholesterol And Recurrent Events (CARE) study. *Circulation* 99:216-223, 1999.

25. Blauw GJ, Lagaay AM, Smelt AH, et al: Stroke, statins, and cholesterol. A meta-analysis of randomized, placebo-controlled, double-blind trials with HMG-CoA reductase inhibitors. *Stroke* 28:946-950, 1997.

26. Belcaro G, Nicolaides AN, Laurora G, et al: Ultrasound morphology classification of the arterial wall and cardiovascular events in a 6-year follow-up study. *Arterioscler Thromb Vasc Biol* 16:851-856, 1996.

27. Hertzer NR, Young JR, Beven EG, et al: Coronary angiography in 506 patients with extracranial cerebrovascular disease. *Arch Intern Med* 145:849-852, 1985.

28. Salenius JP: The course of atherosclerotic diseases after carotid

endarterectomy in 279 patients followed-up for 21 years. *J Intern Med* 225:373-378, 1989.

29. Hertzer NR, Beven EG, Young JR, et al: Coronary artery disease in peripheral vascular patients. A classification of 1000 coronary angiograms and results of surgical management. *Ann Surg* 199:223-233, 1984.

30. Newman AB, Shemanski L, Manolio TA, et al: Ankle-arm index as a predictor of cardiovascular disease and mortality in the Cardiovascular Health Study. The Cardiovascular Health Study Group. *Arterioscler Thromb Vasc Biol* 19:538-545, 1999.

31. O'Riordain DS, O'Donnell JA: Realistic expectations for the patient with intermittent claudication. *Br J Surg* 78:861-863, 1993.

32. Summary of the second report of the National Cholesterol Education Program (NCEP) Expert Panel on Detection, Evaluation, and Treatment of High Blood Cholesterol in Adults (Adult Treatment Panel II). *JAMA* 269:3015-3023, 1993.

PART VI

Basic Science

CHAPTER 15

Molecular Demolition: The Role of Matrix Metalloproteinases in Arterial Disease

Kathleen M. Lewis, BS
Research Fellow, Department of Surgery, University of Nebraska Medical Center, Omaha

Jason P. Rehm, MD
Resident, Department of Surgery, University of Nebraska Medical Center, Omaha

B. Timothy Baxter, MD
Professor of Surgery, Department of Surgery, University of Nebraska Medical Center, Omaha

The basis of many important clinical advances lies in prior discoveries made at the basic science level. The clinical vascular surgeon has a key role in this process, providing the impetus for basic research by identification and characterization of important clinical problems. As clinicians, we have all puzzled over why one patient's carotid stenosis should have a benign clinical course for years while another patient becomes symptomatic with acute progression from moderate- to high-grade stenosis. Why is it that a few small aneurysms grow very rapidly while most grow very little or not at all? The answer to these important clinical questions relates to the local activity of important protein-degrading enzymes that affect the stability of the artery and the atherosclerotic plaque.

The integrity of the large elastic arteries such as the aorta and the carotid artery is dependent on matrix macromolecules, especially, elastin and collagen. These proteins, which are synthesized and maintained by native mesenchymal cells (smooth muscle cells and fibroblasts), provide tensile strength and critically important elastomechanical properties. Additionally, collagen makes up a significant proportion of the atherosclerotic plaque, contributing to both its mass and structural integrity. Elastin and the fibrillar collagens are among the most stable of all known proteins, but they are susceptible to degradation by a family of tightly regulated matrix degrading enzymes called the matrix metalloproteinases (MMPs). Because of the tremendous capacity of these enzymes to destroy structural matrices, loss of control at 1 of 3 important steps governing their activity can lead to arterial injury and plaque instability.

BASIC MMP STRUCTURE

The extensive remodeling that occurs in arterial disease clearly implicates enzymes capable of degrading matrix substrates. The MMPs, also referred to as matrixins, have gained increased attention because of their ability to degrade vital structural components of the vascular wall that are relatively resistant to injury by other proteinases. MMPs are a family of more than 20 structurally related, zinc-dependent endopeptidases that are involved in turnover of the extracellular matrix. They are essential for all processes involving matrix remodeling and are coordinately regulated during normal growth, development, and wound healing.

MMPs can be classified into at least 4 general subfamilies based on the specific substrates of the extracellular matrix that they bind and metabolize. These subfamilies include (1) collagenases that degrade intact fibrillar collagens; (2) stromelysins, which have the broadest substrate specificity degrading proteoglycans, fibronectin, and laminin; (3) gelatinases that hydrolyze denatured fibrillar collagens (hence their name), and degrade basement membrane (type IV) collagen and elastin; and (4) the membrane-type MMPs (MT-MMPs), which are distinguished not by their substrate specificity, but because they have a transmembrane domain that interacts with cellular plasma membrane. Taken together, these MMPs are capable of degrading all the components of the arterial extracellular matrix. Because of the importance of elastin and the fibrillar collagens (type I and III) in the normal artery and in plaque, the collagenases and gelatinases have been the major focus of investigation of aneurysmal disease and atherosclerosis.

Each different MMP has a unique structural sequence, but they all share important functional domains including a signal peptide, propeptide domain, catalytic domain, a hinge region, and a hemopexin or carboxyl domain. The basic elements of some of the MMPs implicated in aneurysmal disease and atherosclerosis are shown in Figure 1. The *signal peptide* can be thought of as a handle that the cell recognizes and uses to transport the protein. It functions by facilitating secretion into the endoplasmic reticulum and export from the cell. The *propeptide* acts as a guard that keeps the active site covered until the MMP is safely transported out of the cell (Fig 2). This prevents the enzyme from degrading or damaging itself or the intracellular structures it contacts during synthesis and secretion. Removal of the propeptide is an important step in extracellular regulation of MMP activity (Fig 3).

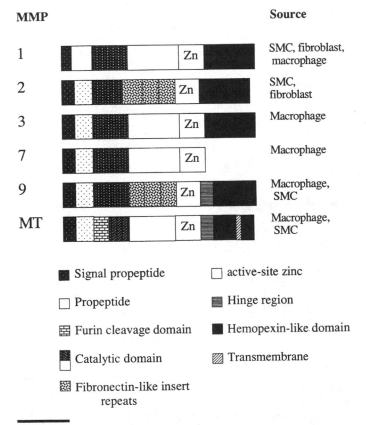

FIGURE 1.
MMP structural domains. The common structural domains found in some of the MMPs implicated in arterial diseases. *Abbreviations: Zn,* zinc; *SMC,* smooth muscle cell; *MT,* membrane-type.

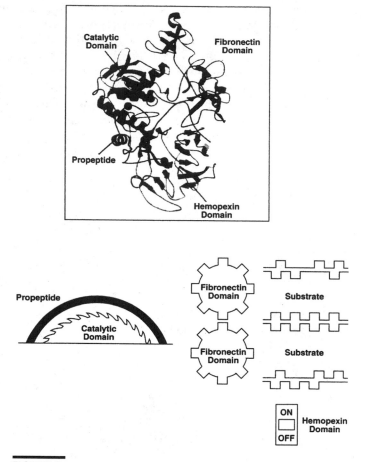

FIGURE 2.

MMP functional domains. The structure of pro-MMP-2 was recently derived using x-ray crystallography. Bottom half is a schematic showing the relationship and role of each functional domain. The propeptide acts as a guard, keeping the active site covered until its activity is required. The fibronectin domains "grab" the substrate. The 3-dimensional structure around the active site and these fibronectin binding sites confer specificity, because only substrates with the appropriate conformation and with corresponding fibronectin binding domains can be bound. The catalytic domain performs the cleavage. The hemopexin domain can help confer specificity by contributing to the 3-dimensional structure of the active site. Additionally, it can be thought of as an on-off switch because it is the binding site for tissue inhibitors of MMPs (TIMPs). TIMPs will inactivate MMPs. (Reprinted with permission from Morgunova E, Tuuttila A, Bergmann U, et al: Structure of human pro-matrix metalloproteinase-2: Activation mechanism revealed. *Science* 284:1667-1670. Copyright 1999, American Association for the Advancement of Science.)

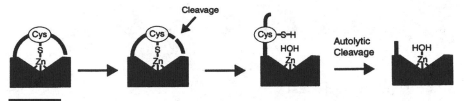

FIGURE 3.
MMP activation. The proenzyme prevents association of the active site with a water molecule. Stepwise activation of MMPs occurs after initial cleavage, which takes place in an exposed region ("bait region") of the proenzyme, resulting in an intermediate form of the MMP. This intermediate then autolytically cleaves the remainder of the proenzyme, resulting in the fully active form of the MMP. (Adapted from Sato H, Seiki M: Membrane-type matrix metalloproteinases [MT-MMPs] in tumor metastasis. *J Biochem [Tokyo]* 119:209-215, 1996.)

The *catalytic domain* performs the proteolytic cleavage of the substrate. It is connected to the adjacent hemopexin domain by a linker or a *hinge region*. The *hemopexin or carboxyl terminus domain* contributes to a groove in the catalytic domain created by the fibronectin repeats. Thus, it could have a role in determining which substrates fit into the active site for cleavage. Additionally, the domain can be thought of as the on-off switch for the MMP because it is the binding site for tissue inhibitors of MMPs (TIMPs). The binding of a TIMP molecule to this domain will inhibit or inactivate the MMP.

REGULATION OF MMPS

The regulation of MMPs occurs at 3 levels: (1) gene transcription, (2) conversion of the inactive zymogen precursor to the active form of the enzyme, and (3) inhibition by endogenous tissue inhibitors (Fig 4).

TRANSCRIPTIONAL REGULATION

The signal for the cell to begin to make copies of messenger RNA to increase production of the MMP protein is regulated by a variety of local factors including inflammatory cytokines, growth factors, cellular transformation, and hormones.[1] MMP synthesis can also be modulated through integrin-mediated changes in cell shape.[1] Other possible controls, such as changes in the stability of the mRNA or its efficiency of translation into protein, may also be operative.

ACTIVATION OF MMPS

MMPs are synthesized as preproenzymes, and most are processed to and secreted as inactive proenzymes. The exception may be the

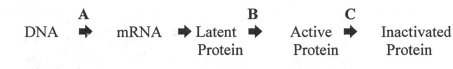

A-transcriptional regulation
cytokines, growth factors, hormones,
changes in cell morphology

B–activation of proenzyme
plasmin, trypsin, neutrophil
elastase, MMPs

C-inactivation of enzyme
TIMP, alpha-2 macroglobulin

FIGURE 4.
MMP regulation occurs at 3 levels. MMP synthesis is controlled at the transcriptional level **(A)** by a variety of soluble mediators and changes in cell morphology. Latent MMPs are converted to their active form **(B)** by other proteolytic enzymes including serine proteinases and other MMPs. Inhibitors may bind and inactivate **(C)** the fully active MMP molecule.

membrane-type family of MMPs that contains a furin recognition site. Furin is an enzyme that activates proteins within the cell. The extracellular activation of all other MMPs is one of the critical steps leading to extracellular matrix breakdown. The latency of MMPs is caused by the N-terminal domain of the prodomain that protrudes into the active site (Fig 3).[2] This prevents the association of a water molecule with the zinc atom, which is necessary for the catalytic activity of the enzyme. The propeptide is cleaved sequentially, with the initial cleavage typically taking place in an exposed "bait" region that is recognized by many serine proteinases such as plasmin, trypsin, and neutrophil elastase. The bait region may also be recognized by MMP-3 or MT-MMPs to start the activation process.[3]

TISSUE INHIBITORS OF MMPS
The action of MMPs is also regulated through inhibition by endogenous specific tissue inhibitors of the MMPs, the TIMPs.[1] In normal tissues, the TIMPs counterbalance the activity of the MMPs by binding in a 1:1 molar stoichiometry. The exact mechanism by

which the TIMPs inhibit MMPs is not well understood, but most likely this involves some alteration or interaction with the MMP active site. One surprising twist in the role of TIMP has been its requirement for activation of MMP-2. TIMP-2 is required in low concentrations for binding and activation of MMP-2 by MT1-MMP at the cell surface, whereas at higher concentrations, TIMP binding inhibits active MMP-2.[4] α_2-Macroglobulin is another physiologic inhibitor of activated MMPs.

ABDOMINAL AORTIC ANEURYSM

All vascular surgeons are keenly aware that abdominal aortic aneurysm (AAA) is a common and potentially deadly disease affecting at least 2% of the US population. This disease is the primary cause of approximately 15,000 deaths per year in the United States alone,[5] and there is evidence that the incidence of AAA among the elderly may be increasing. Among those affected, the only therapy proven to alter the natural history of the disease is aneurysmorrhaphy. Because most AAAs detected in screening studies are small and there is no therapy to inhibit their growth, general screening programs for AAA have not been endorsed. Clearly, screening would become routine if there were an effective therapy that inhibited the progression of small AAAs.

The aorta is the largest of the elastic arteries, performing 2 important functions: it acts as a conduit transporting blood from the heart to the rest of the body, and it reduces cardiac workload by absorbing energy as blood is ejected from the heart. These functions require that the aortic wall possess both tensile strength and elasticity, properties conferred largely by the matrix proteins, collagen and elastin. These proteins are synthesized and maintained by the resident mesenchymal cells (smooth muscle cells [SMCs] and fibroblasts) in a highly regulated fashion designed to maintain the functional integrity of the vascular wall. However, the ability to synthesize functional elastin fibers is lost or greatly diminished after birth. Thus, when elastin-containing tissues such as the aorta are injured, the reparative process results in tissue with altered biomechanical properties.

Studies investigating the pathogenesis of aneurysm formation have demonstrated marked changes in the normal orderly lamellar structure of the aortic wall. One of the most striking histologic features of aneurysmal tissue is the fragmentation of the medial elastin. There is a large decrease in the relative elastin concentration that results both from the redistribution of elastin over a larger surface area and dilution by the synthesis of large amounts of fibrillar collagen. The collagen synthesis occurs, presumably, as part of an ongoing attempt at repair.[6,7]

PROTEOLYSIS IN AAA

The matrix destruction associated with AAA has focused on a relatively limited number of enzymes. AAA tissue has been examined for the presence of both elastolytic and collagenolytic enzymes. The elastolytic enzymes found in AAA include MMP–9[8-10] and MMP-12.[11] The collagenase, MMP-1, is also present in AAA tissues. We have been particularly interested in MMP-2 because its ability to degrade both elastin and fibrillar collagen is unique. We have found both increased levels and an increase in the activated form of MMP-2 in AAA tissues.[12]

Another important histologic feature of AAA tissues is a remarkably intense inflammatory cell infiltrate. These inflammatory cells produce MMPs (MMP-1, MMP-9, and MMP-12) and regulate the expression of these enzymes by local mesenchymal cells (MMP-1 and MMP-2 produced by SMC and fibroblasts). The presence of macrophages and lymphocytes in AAA tissue and their spatial association with expressed MMPs suggest a central role in regulation of individual MMPs. These descriptive studies of AAA tissue have provided a useful starting point for investigating MMPs in AAA, but they are limited in their ability to show a direct "cause and effect" relationship. Recent studies using animal models of AAA have, however, established a mechanistic link between MMPs and aneurysm pathogenesis and progression.

ANIMAL MODELS

Two experimental aneurysm models lend strong support to the theory that the marked inflammation noted in AAA plays an etiologic role. Gertz et al[13] have found that aneurysms can be created in the rabbit carotid artery by inducing a transmural inflammatory response through application of calcium chloride to the adventitia. We have used this model to create AAAs in mice. In developing another widely used AAA model, Anidjar et al[14] have shown that elastase infusion under superphysiologic pressures produces aneurysms in the aorta. The theoretical basis for this model was direct elastin degradation, but in fact, the dilatation showed a temporal correlation, not with the early elastin degradation, but with the ensuing inflammatory response.[15] Ricci et al[16] provided corroborative evidence for the key role of inflammation in this model by demonstrating decreased aortic dilatation when leukocyte adhesion was blocked by an antibody to CD18. These models suggest that the inflammatory infiltrate, and not direct elastin injury by calcium chloride or elastase, is primarily responsible for aortic dilatation.

Further characterization of these models suggests that the role of inflammatory cells in the pathogenesis of AAA may relate to their ability to regulate proteolysis. Additional characterization of the elastase infusion model has shown that the inflammatory cell infiltration is accompanied by an increase in MMP-2 and MMP-9.[17] Of note, a nonspecific MMP inhibitor, doxycycline, inhibited aneurysm formation in this model.[17] Holmes et al[18] also investigated the role of the inflammatory cascade in this model by blocking arachidonic acid metabolite production with indomethacin, inhibiting both MMP production and aneurysm formation. Perhaps the most compelling argument for the role of MMPs in AAA was a study demonstrating that local overexpression of TIMP by transfected SMCs inhibited aneurysm formation in a transplant model of AAA.[19] Unlike doxycycline, which is a nonspecific MMP inhibitor, TIMP is highly specific in its inhibition of MMPs. Taken together, these studies suggest that increased local MMP activity has a pivotal role in aneurysm formation and progression.

FUTURE DIRECTION

This work has led to planning of clinical trials with a goal of inhibiting progression of small AAAs. Animal studies have suggested several approaches that could work: (1) local inhibition of MMP production or (2) inhibition of the inflammatory response. A variety of hydoxamate-type MMP inhibitors, which work by reversibly chelating the zinc ion at the active site, are in clinical trials for neoplastic diseases based on evidence that cancer cells use MMPs for invasion and neovascularity. The tetracycline derivatives inhibit MMPs, a property independent of their antibiotic moiety. Because of the extensive clinical experience and their safety profile, tetracycline derivatives will be an obvious target for clinical trials. As these trials are planned, it is important to keep in mind that animal models of aneurysms cannot precisely replicate the pathogenesis of chronic AAAs. Experience has taught us that extrapolating from animal models can be fraught with problems and unexpected outcomes. It will be important, therefore, that any pharmacologic agents given to inhibit AAA growth be used, initially, in controlled trials.

ROLE OF MMPS IN PLAQUE RUPTURE

The process of plaque rupture has gained increased attention as vascular surgeons, cardiologists, and cardiovascular researchers have recognized its role as an underlying cause of stroke and acute coronary syndromes.[20,21] Despite favorable trends in coronary artery disease in the United States, cerebral vascular disease is increasing in incidence. Furthermore, it is predicted that within 20 years, ischemic heart disease could surpass infectious disease as the leading cause of death worldwide.[22]

PLAQUE COMPOSITION

Atherosclerotic plaque is the result of complex interactions between resident cells in the vessel wall, including SMCs and endothelial cells, and infiltrating immune cells.[21] Plaque development is predominantly an asymptomatic process until a hemodynamically significant stenosis develops. This typically occurs when the arterial diameter is reduced by at least 50% with a corresponding 75% decrease in lumen area. At this point, the clinical syndrome of reduced blood flow through the affected artery may remain stable for years.[22] However, in other instances, the structural integrity of the plaque is diminished, and plaque rupture results in acute occlusion or arterial embolization.

The basic architecture of plaque is highly characteristic: the central core is composed of extracellular lipids and debris that is surrounded by a cap made of collagenous tissue. This fibrous tissue gives the plaque its structural integrity. Different stages of plaque development are associated with differing ratios of lipid and fibrous tissue; the early plaque contains little or no extracellular lipid.[20,21] Conversely, late-stage complex plaque contains a much greater proportion of lipid with relatively little fibrous tissue. Thus, the ratio of fibrous tissue to lipid can vary widely, and plaques with varying morphologies can be found in different locations within a patient.[20]

PLAQUE STABILITY

Changes in 2 important features of plaque signal progression toward an unstable lesion. The first of these is a change in plaque composition. The loss of fibrous collagen and a relative increase in lipid leads to instability. This is accompanied by a change in cellularity, with decreasing numbers of collagen-producing SMCs and increasing inflammatory cells.[23] These changes in cellular makeup also correlate with decreasing plaque stability. This loss of structural integrity renders the plaque susceptible to the mechanical forces constantly exerted by blood in the lumen. The correlation between plaque type, content (lipid vs collagen), and cellular composition (SMC vs macrophages) are shown in Table 1.

TABLE 1.
Plaque Composition and Cellularity

	Group A	Group B	Group C
Lipid core (% plaque area)	12.7	27.3	56.7
Cell number per mm^2			
Mφ in cap	60	79	142
SMC in cap	183	186	60
Mφ in shoulder	96	108	153
SMC in shoulder	183	212	113
Ratio SMC:Mφ in cap tissue	8:1	4:1	1:1

Group A, intact plaques containing no thrombosis; Group B, intact plaques with thrombus; Group C, ulcerated plaques.
Abbreviations: Mφ, Macrophages; *SMC,* smooth muscle cells.
(Adapted from Davies MJ, Richardson PD, Woolf N, et al: Risk of thrombosis in human atherosclerotic plaques: Role of extracellular lipid, macrophage, and smooth muscle cell content. *Br Heart J* 69:377-381, 1993.)

As suggested above, the increased prominence of the lipid core in the vulnerable plaque gives way to reduced rigidity of the tissue and thus an increased chance of rupture of the fibrous cap. Mechanical forces that may contribute to rupture include shear stress injury, transient collapse of the stenotic lesion, and rupture of the vasa vasorum.[22] In studying human plaque morphology, Cheng et al[24] found that 10 of 12 ruptures occurred within 15 degrees of areas of high sheer stress predicted by computer modeling. The regions of the plaque predisposed to intimal rupture caused by high sheer stress are the shoulder and the center of the plaque (Fig 5). Because plaque is a heterogeneous material, however, rupture may be found at other sites. Interestingly, the highest relative density of inflammatory cells is found in these rupture-prone areas,[25] suggesting that there are signaling mechanisms in the plaque for macrophage recruitment to areas of greatest shear stress. Macrophages are activated in the plaque by oxidized low-density lipoprotein. These activated cells are capable of secreting a host of proteolytic enzymes including serine proteases, cysteine proteases, and MMPs.[22]

MMPS IN ATHEROMA

The hypothesis that MMPs could be involved in atherosclerosis and plaque stability was tested initially by comparing the MMP content in normal and atherosclerotic arteries. Increased levels of

MMP-1, MMP-3, MMP-7, and MMP-9 were found in diseased tissue compared with modest expression in normal arteries. This result is not unexpected considering that these MMPs are secreted by activated macrophages, which are abundant in atherosclerotic tissue and not generally present in the normal artery. By immunohistochemistry, these macrophage-associated MMPs localize to the fibrous cap and the shoulders of the plaque[26] with the exception of MMP-7, which is found around the lipid core (Fig 6). MMP-2 is an SMC product expressed at equivalent levels in both normal and atherosclerotic arteries.[26] MMP expression can also be found in association with other cells, especially endothelial cells overlying the plaque and in the microvessels around the plaque.[26]

The expression of the direct MMP antagonists, the tissue inhibitors of MMP (TIMP-1, TIMP-2, and TIMP–3), has been found in both normal and diseased tissue. The spatial distribution of the cells that express these TIMPs seems to correlate with expression of their MMP counterpart.[26] TIMP-1 is a macrophage product that binds and inhibits the macrophages' MMP products. TIMP-2 inhibits MMP-2 and is secreted by mesenchymal cells. The close proximity of the enzyme and the inhibitor lends support to the idea that the TIMPs play an important regulatory role in restraining pathologic MMP activity.[26]

MMP-2 is found primarily in association with the mesenchymal cells of the media and adventitia. These cells have the capacity to

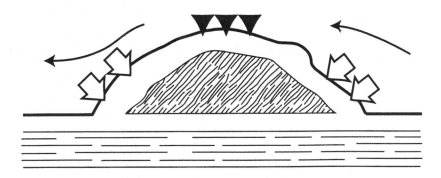

FIGURE 5.
Site of plaque rupture. An isolated plaque is shown in the artery wall. Certain regions of the plaque are predisposed to plaque rupture caused by high mechanical stress. The "cap" *(darkened arrowheads)* is the site at which nearly one third (30%) of all plaque ruptures take place. Approximately one half (49%) of plaque ruptures take place in the shoulder region *(open arrows).*[32] Because of its heterogeneity, the remaining ruptures occur at varying sites.

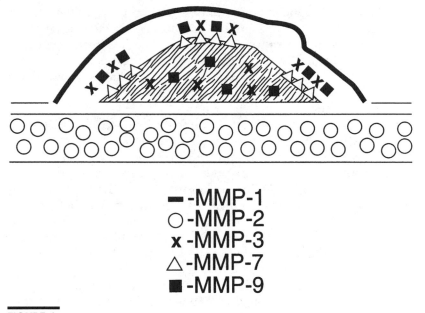

- -MMP-1
○ -MMP-2
x -MMP-3
△ -MMP-7
■ -MMP-9

FIGURE 6.
MMP localization in plaque. MMPs are expressed in different areas of the plaque. MMP-1 is concentrated in the endothelial cells overlying the plaque. MMP-2 is found in the medial smooth muscle cells, whereas MMP-3 and MMP-9 are present in the rupture-prone cap and shoulder regions. MMP-7 is found primarily in the macrophages overlying the lipid core.

produce significantly more MMP-1 and MMP-2 than macrophages.[27] Although there is no significant elevation of MMP-2 in the diseased artery, there is significant activation of the MMP-2 found in plaque. MMP-2 is uniquely activated at the cell surface in association with MT-MMPs. Recent work by Rajavashisth et al[28] has shown that among the family of 4 known MT-MMPs, MT1-MMP is the physiologic activator of MMP-2. Interestingly, this active MMP-2 appears to be bound to matrix by fibronectin binding domains, suggesting direct involvement in matrix destruction.[12]

TREATMENT

The goal of successful treatment of an existent atheroma is to maintain stability of the fibrous sheath protecting the lipid core. One obvious therapeutic consideration is the inhibition of MMPs directly as a step to stabilize plaque. Potent hydroxamate MMP inhibitors are currently being tested as chemotherapeutic agents for cancer. One potential downside to this approach is progressive fibrosis that could inhibit homeostatic MMP activity associated with normal turnover of collagen. This has been clinically apparent with short-term use in the tendon sheaths where some patients lose mobility of their hands, a process that is reversed when the drug dosage is decreased. Of greater concern is fibrosis of other organs such as the liver or lungs.

As with AAA, the tetracycline derivatives also offer potential in treating atherosclerosis. In a recent study, the use of tetracycline derivatives or quinilones within 3 years was associated with a reduced incidence of new myocardial infarction in a recent large cohort trial.[29] Other antibiotics including macrolides (erythromycin), sulfonamides, penicillins, or cephalosporins were not effective. The efficacy of the tetracycline derivatives and quinolones was ascribed to their antibiotic properties against *Chlamydia pneumoniae*. The efficacy of quinolones against *C pneumoniae* is not well documented, and a subsequent trial using newer macrolides, which are highly effective against *C pneumoniae*, showed no benefit.[30] When these studies are considered together, another, perhaps even more plausible explanation for the effectiveness of the tetracycline derivatives comes to mind; their MMP inhibitory properties.

Anti-inflammatory strategies for stabilizing plaque have been used successfully for years without appreciating that this was the operative mechanism. The efficacy of aspirin in preventing adverse cardiovascular and cerebrovascular events has long been attributed to aspirin's anticoagulant properties. As a marker of systemic inflammation, C-reactive protein levels among 543 healthy men were found to correlate with the risk of subsequent myocardial infarction and ischemic stroke.[31] The risk of these events was reduced by more than 50% among those with the highest C-reactive protein levels who took aspirin. These data strongly suggest that the beneficial effects of aspirin in reducing cardiac and cerebral vascular events are related to aspirin's anti-inflammatory properties. Whether this reduction in inflammation will be found to correlate with a reduction in local MMP activity is not known but seems likely, given the ability of proinflammatory cytokines to upregulate MMPs.

CONCLUSIONS

The practicing vascular surgeon has helped to define and characterize several common and dangerous clinical syndromes that result, in part, from local overexpression of proteolytic enzymes.

At the basic science level, animal models are being developed to elucidate the molecular mechanisms of these disease processes. Trials to inhibit the growth of small AAAs are being planned and these therapies, if successful, may be widely used within the next 5 years. MMPs appear to play a central role in the loss of plaque stability. The role of MMPs in restenosis is only now being studied. It is likely that MMP inhibitors will become an important part of the medical treatment of patients with aneurysms and atherosclerosis. Because of your role in providing primary care for patients with peripheral or cerebrovascular atherosclerosis and aneurysms, you the vascular surgeon will have a role in the clinical investigation and implementation of these advances in the clinics and at the bedside.

REFERENCES

1. Nagase H: Section matrix metalloproteinases, in Hooper N (ed): *Zinc Metalloproteases in Health and Disease,* ed. London, Taylor & Francis, 1996.
2. Becker JW, Marcy AI, Rokosz LL, et al: Stromelysin-1: Three-dimensional structure of the inhibited catalytic domain and of the C-truncated proenzyme. *Protein Sci* 4:1966-1976, 1995.
3. Woessner JF Jr: Matrix metalloproteinases and their inhibitors in connective tissue remodeling. *FASEB J* 5:2145-2154, 1991.
4. Butler GS, Butler MJ, Atkinson SJ, et al: The TIMP2 membrane type 1 metalloproteinase "receptor" regulates the concentration and efficient activation of progelatinase A. A kinetic study. *J Biol Chem* 273:871-880, 1998.
5. National Center for Health Statistics, Graves E: Detailed diagnoses and procedures, National Hospital Discharge Survey. *Vital Health Stat* 13(107):91-1768, 1991.
6. Rizzo RJ, McCarthy WJ, Dixit SN, et al: Collagen types and matrix protein content in human abdominal aortic aneurysms. *J Vasc Surg* 10:365-373, 1989.
7. Baxter BT, McGee GS, Shively VP, et al: Elastin content, cross-links, and mRNA in normal and aneurysmal human aorta. *J Vasc Surg* 16:192-200, 1992.
8. Herron GS, Unemori E, Wong M, et al: Connective tissue proteinases and inhibitors in abdominal aortic aneurysms. Involvement of the vasa vasorum in the pathogenesis of aortic aneurysms. *Arterioscler Thromb* 11:1667-1677, 1991.
9. Newman KM, Ogata Y, Malon AM, et al: Identification of matrix metalloproteinases 3 (stromelysin-1) and 9 (gelatinase B) in abdominal aortic aneurysm. *Arterioscler Thromb* 14:1315-1320,1994.
10. Thompson RW, Holmes DR, Mertens RA, et al: Production and localization of 92-kilodalton gelatinase in abdominal aortic aneurysms. An

elastolytic metalloproteinase expressed by aneurysm-infiltrating macrophages. *J Clin Invest* 96:318-326, 1995.

11. Curci JA, Liao S, Huffman MD, et al: Expression and localization of macrophage elastase (matrix metalloproteinase-12) in abdominal aortic aneurysms. *J Clin Invest* 102:1900-1910, 1998.

12. Davis VPR, Baca-Regen L, Yoshifumi I, et al: Matrix metalloproteinase-2 production and its binding to the matrix are increased in abdominal aortic aneurysms. *Arterioscler Thromb Vasc Biol* 18:1625-1633, 1998.

13. Gertz SD, Kurgan A, Eisenberg D: Aneurysm of the rabbit common carotid artery induced by periarterial application of calcium chloride in vivo. *J Clin Invest* 81:649-656, 1988.

14. Anidjar S, Salzmann JL, Gentric D, et al: Elastase-induced experimental aneurysms in rats. *Circulation* 82:973-981, 1990.

15. Anidjar S, Dobrin PB, Eichorst M, et al: Correlation of inflammatory infiltrate with the enlargement of experimental aortic aneurysms. *J Vasc Surg* 16:139-147, 1992.

16. Ricci MA, Strindberg G, Slaiby JM, et al: Anti-CD 18 monoclonal antibody slows experimental aortic aneurysm expansion. *J Vasc Surg* 23:301-307, 1996.

17. Petrinec D, Liao S, Holmes DR, et al: Doxycycline inhibition of aneurysmal degeneration in an elastase-induced rat model of abdominal aortic aneurysm: Preservation of aortic elastin associated with suppressed production of 92 kD gelatinase. *J Vasc Surg* 23:336-346, 1996.

18. Holmes DR, Petrinec D, Wester W, et al: Indomethacin prevents elastase-induced abdominal aortic aneurysms in the rat. *J Surg Res* 63:305-309, 1996.

19. Allaire E, Forough R, Clowes M, et al: Local overexpression of TIMP-1 prevents aortic aneurysm degeneration and rupture in a rat model. *J Clin Invest* 102:1413-1420, 1998.

20. Gutstein DE, Fuster V: Pathophysiology and clinical significance of atherosclerotic plaque rupture. *Cardiovasc Res* 41:323-333, 1999.

21. van der Wal AC: Atherosclerotic plaque rupture: Pathologic basis of plaque stability and instability. *Cardiovasc Res* 41:334-344, 1999.

22. Arroyo LH, Lee RT: Mechanisms of plaque rupture: Mechanical and biologic interactions. *Cardiovasc Res* 41:369-375, 1999.

23. Bauriedel G, Hutter R, Welsch U, et al: Role of smooth muscle cell death in advanced coronary primary lesions: Implications for plaque instability. *Cardiovasc Res* 41:480-488, 1999.

24. Cheng GC, Loree HM, Kamm RD, et al: Distribution of circumferential stress in ruptured and stable atherosclerotic lesions. A structural analysis with histopathological correlation. *Circulation* 87:1179-1187, 1993.

25. Davies MJ, Richardson PD, Woolf N, et al: Risk of thrombosis in human atherosclerotic plaques: Role of extracellular lipid, macrophage, and smooth muscle cell content. *Br Heart J* 69:377-381, 1993.

26. Fabunmi RP, Libby P: Regulation of metalloproteinases and their

inhibitors in atheroma, in Valentin Fuster M (ed): *The Vulnerable Atherosclerotic Plaque: Understanding, Identification, and Modification*, ed 1. Armonk, NY, Futura Publishing, 1999, pp 365-381.

27. Welgus HG, Campbell EJ, Cury JD, et al: Neutral metalloproteinases produced by human mononuclear phagocytes. Enzyme profile, regulation, and expression during cellular development. *J Clin Invest* 86:1496-1502, 1990.

28. Rajavashisth TB, Xu XP, Jovinge S, et al: Membrane type 1 matrix metalloproteinase expression in human atherosclerotic plaques: Evidence for activation by proinflammatory mediators. *Circulation* 99:3103-3109, 1999.

29. Meier CR, Derby LE, Jick SS, et al: Antibiotics and risk of subsequent first-time acute myocardial infarction [see comments]. *JAMA* 281:427-431, 1999.

30. Anderson JL, Muhlestein JB, Carlquist J, et al: Randomized secondary prevention trial of azithromycin in patients with coronary artery disease and serological evidence for *Chlamydia pneumoniae* infection: The Azithromycin in Coronary Artery Disease: Elimination of Myocardial Infection with Chlamydia (ACADEMIC) study [see comments]. *Circulation* 99:1540-1547, 1999.

31. Ridker PM, Cushman M, Stampfer MJ, et al: Inflammation, aspirin, and the risk of cardiovascular disease in apparently healthy men [see comments]. *N Engl J Med* 336:973-979, 1997. (Published erratum appears in *N Engl J Med* 337:356, 1997.)

32. Richardson PD, Davies MJ, Born GVR: Influence of plaque configuration and stress distribution on fissuring of coronary atherosclerotic plaques. *Lancet* 2:941-944, 1989.

CHAPTER 16

Regulation of Angiogenesis: Mechanisms and Clinical Implications

Michael T. Watkins, MD
Associate Professor of Surgery, Departments of Surgery, Pathology, and Laboratory Medicine, Boston University School of Medicine, Co-chief of Surgical Services, VAMC Boston, Massachusetts

Charles F. Bratton, MD
Chief Surgical Resident, Department of Surgery, Boston Medical Center, Boston University School of Medicine, Massachusetts

Therapeutic angiogenesis is an exciting frontier within the management of a variety of ischemic and proliferative clinical disorders. Clinical applications of research on angiogenesis have involved the quantitation of angiogenesis for use in diagnosis and prognosis, the acceleration of angiogenesis during repair, and the inhibition of angiogenesis. One form of therapeutic angiogenesis is a strategy whereby one of the known specific angiogenic factors is delivered to the ischemic region of a targeted organ. A desirable end point of this form of therapeutic angiogenesis would be to promote new collateral vessels to ischemic myocardium, leg muscles, and other tissues. Pharmacologic interventions to modulate the function of ischemic organs have failed to alter the fundamental problem—inadequate blood flow. Conceptually, therapeutic angiogenesis would provide the most direct, relevant approach to alleviating the imbalance between supply and demand of blood. Therapeutic strategies to *inhibit* angiogenesis have been sought since Folkman et al[1] observed that tumor cells could not grow beyond 2 to 3 mm without developing new blood vessels. The central therapeutic concept that evolved as a result of this observation is that inhibition of blood vessel growth might control or prevent tumor growth, metastasis, or both. This chapter reviews the evolution of the field of therapeutic angiogenesis, taking into account the rich basic scientific foundation of this emerging field, and places current clinical trials in perspective.

ROOTS OF THERAPEUTIC ANGIOGENESIS

The term "angiogenesis" was first coined in 1935 to describe the formation of new blood vessels in the placenta.[1] Angiogenesis, strictly defined, is a process that leads to generation of new blood vessels from pre-existing ones. The process of angiogenesis differs from vasculogenesis, in which endothelial cell (EC) precursors called angioblasts associate to form early vessel tubes. Tissues that are vascularized in this fashion are generally of endodermal origin and include the pancreas, lung, spleen, heart, and dorsal aorta.[2] In contrast, angiogenesis appears to be the sole means of neovascularization during processes such as wound healing. Tissues of ectodermal and mesodermal origin, such as kidney and brain, are vascularized by angiogenesis. Endothelial cells are important components of the vasculature whose proliferation appears to be stringently controlled. Labeling studies have documented that the turnover rate of vascular ECs in normal tissues of adults is low, with 0.01% to 0.1% of the large- and small-vessel ECs labeled after a 24-hour ^{3}H-thymidine pulse.[3] Because of this low proliferation rate, the phenomenon of angiogenesis was largely inaccessible to conventional experimental techniques. Investigators believed that an understanding of angiogenesis was essential to develop strategies which could potentiate wound healing and the treatment of ischemic tissues, and perhaps inhibit the growth of tumors. In the mid 1970s, four techniques were developed to study angiogenesis:

1. The corneal micropocket technique permitted linear measurement of individual capillaries as they grew toward a tumor or an angiogenic substance implanted in the rabbit,[4] mouse, or rat cornea.
2. Biocompatible polymers were developed for the sustained release of angiogenic factors in vivo.
3. The chick embryo chorioallantoic membrane was used to detect angiogenic activity of partially purified fractions from tumor extracts.[5]
4. Vascular ECs were cultured from aortic,[6] venous,[7] and capillary tissues[8] and used to guide the purification of EC growth factors.

Angiogenesis in vivo does not occur in isolation with just one cell type present. For this reason, some investigators have set up coculture models of angiogenesis in which ECs are grown in the presence of other cells that can promote angiogenesis. Specifically, cancer cells, keratinocytes, and astroglial cells may be studied with endothelium in coculture systems. In these coculture systems, some of the proangiogenic stimuli can be provided by a soluble factor; in other cases, cell-cell contact is needed. These models provide a mechanism to study the importance of cell-cell communication and its disruption in angiogenesis. In most in vivo models, it is difficult to differentiate between inflammatory and angiogenic activities separately. Despite these experimental problems, several well-defined angiogenic peptide growth factors have been well characterized (Table 1).

Among the first growth factors to be described were basic fibroblast growth factor (bFGF) isolated from brain[9] and EC growth factor (ECGF) isolated from hypothalamus.[10] Retina,[11] eye,[12] and cartilage[13] were also identified as sources of ECGFs. A significant breakthrough in this field developed as a result of the observation that an ECGF derived from rat chondrosarcoma had a marked affinity for heparin. Heparin affinity chromatography was used to

TABLE 1.

Angiogenic Growth Factors and Inhibitors

Proangiogenic Factors	Angiogenic Inhibitors
Fibroblast growth factors (1, 2)	Angiostatin
Vascular endothelial cell growth factor	Endostatin
Transforming growth factor–β	Thrombospondin
Angiogenin	Platelet factor 4
Interleukin-8	Prolactin
Proliferin	Placenta proliferin-related peptide
Prostaglandins (PGE)	Metalloproteinase inhibitors
Placenta growth factor	Interleukin-12
Granulocyte colony stimulating factor	
Platelet-derived growth factor	
Platelet-derived endothelial cell growth factor	
Hepatocyte growth factor	

achieve a rapid purification of a homogeneous, cationic, 18 kd molecular weight EC mitogen.[14] The chondrosarcoma-derived factor was angiogenic in both chick embryo and rat cornea bioassays. This purification process led to isolation of a number of angiogenic polypeptides. By 1985, the primary amino acid structures of 2 heparin-binding growth factors—bFGF,[15] a 146–amino acid polypeptide, and acidic FGF (aFGF),[16] a 140–amino acid polypeptide—had been determined. Both bFGF and aFGF were found to be structurally related, having a 53% absolute sequence homology. The FGFs constitute a larger family of at least 18 structurally related polypeptides. The FGF prototypes FGF-1 (aFGF) and FGF-2 (bFGF) are unique because neither possesses a classic signal sequence[17] to direct its secretion through the endoplasmic reticulum–Golgi apparatus. This feature contrasts with the presence of a functional signal sequence within the structure of the remaining FGF family members.

A major breakthrough in understanding how FGF–1 is secreted was demonstrated by Carreira et al.[18] These investigators showed that FGF-1 exists in association with synaptotagmin, a transmembrane component of synaptic vesicles involved in the regulation of organelle traffic and S100A13, a calcium-binding protein. Antisense synaptotagmin–1 gene repressed the release of FGF-1 in response to heat shock. Amlexanox, an anti-inflammatory agent that binds S100A13, also repressed FGF-1 and synaptotagmin release in a dose-dependent manner. These data suggest that the FGF-1 release pathway may be accessible to pharmacologic regulation.

FGF-2 is synthesized by many vascular cells including macrophages, monocytes, fibroblasts, ECs, and vascular smooth muscle. Four different FGF receptors have been characterized, each with a transmembrane domain linked to an intracellular tyrosine kinase. Ligand binding initiates sequential phosphorylation and activation of intracellular signals, resulting in gene transcription and vascular cell proliferation. FGF-2 also upregulates expression of plasminogen activator and integrins critical for cellular migration and luminal formation.

In 1989, vascular permeability factor, previously found to induce vascular leakage in guinea pig skin, was found to have pronounced angiogenic responses in a variety of in vivo models.[19,20] Over the years, several structurally related molecules have been identified, including placenta growth factor, vascular endothelial growth factor-B (VEGF-B), VEGF-C, and VEGF-D. There is compelling evidence that VEGF[4] plays an essential role in the development and differentiation of the cardiovascular system, and the loss of a single VEGF allele results in early lethality in mouse embryos.[21] In vitro, VEGF induces endothelial sprouting from rat aortic rings embedded in a collagen gel. VEGF and FGF-2 demonstrate a potent synergy in their ability to promote angiogenesis in an in vitro model system.[22] VEGF also functions as a survival factor for cultured ECs in serum-depleted conditions, and induces expression of anti-apoptotic proteins Bcl-2 and A1 in human ECs. This potent peptide also induces expression of the serine proteases urokinase-type and tissue-type plasminogen activators in bovine microvascular cells,[23] and stimulates expression of the metalloproteinase interstitial collagenase in human umbilical vein ECs. The vascular leakage and the proteins induced by VEGF facilitate EC migration and proliferation in vivo, providing a crucial step in angiogenesis associated with tumors and wounds. Furthermore, VEGF is believed to be an essential mediator of pathologic angiogenesis associated with ischemic retinal diseases.

It is evident that many angiogenic growth factors stimulate EC proliferation and migration. EC migration is dependent on dissolution and remodeling of the extracellular matrix. Plasminogen activator is a well-characterized proteolytic enzyme of EC origin. Urokinase plasminogen activator is secreted as a proenzyme, which binds to its receptor. The ligand-receptor complex converts plasminogen to plasmin, which actively degrades matrix proteins including fibrin, fibronectin, and laminin. Plasmin activates other proteolytic enzymes, thereby ensuring remodeling within the matrix via metalloproteinases and elastase. EC migration is also dependent on expression of membrane adhesion molecules, termed integrins. Integrins are transmembrane glycoproteins that mediate interaction between cells and the extracellular matrix. The $\alpha v \beta 3$ integrin is a marker of angiogenesis. Monoclonal antibodies to this integrin result in a decrease in tumor-associated blood vessel density. This particular integrin also functions as the EC receptor for fibrin and fibronectin, thereby promoting extracellular matrix formation.

TOOLS FOR EXPERIMENTAL ANGIOGENIC THERAPY: DELIVERY SYSTEMS

There are 2 basic delivery strategies, protein and gene therapy, to achieve benefit. Protein-based therapy is designed to deliver one of the known angiogenic factors to targeted tissue in recombinant protein form. Although there are reports of angiogenesis induced by single administration of a peptide growth factor, most studies of angiogenesis in the heart have used some means of sustained peptide delivery. Sustained delivery techniques have included a number of indwelling catheters (reservoir based) and other infusion techniques including sustained release polymers and biological substrates that are impregnated with growth factor and then implanted into target tissue. Protein-based therapy has the advantage of eliciting minimal immune response, thereby avoiding all the potential complications of inflammation associated with both humoral and cellular immunity.

In contrast, gene therapy is the delivery of the gene encoding for the angiogenic protein with an appropriate transfer vector. Vectors for gene therapy have included naked plasmid cDNA and replication-deficient viral vectors, including adeno-associated virus (AAV), retrovirus, and adenovirus. The plasmid is a genetically engineered, circular, double-stranded DNA molecule containing an expression cassette (the gene to be transferred with an appropriate promotor) and a stop signal. By most estimates, only 0.1% of the plasmid delivered actually reaches the nucleus, and therefore, large quantities of plasmid are required to be delivered to a target organ to achieve effect. There is little if any immune response to plasmid. In contrast, viruses provide an extremely efficient method to transfer replicating and nonreplicating cells. Adenovirus (Ad) is a 36-kilobase (kb) double-stranded DNA virus that transfers genes to a variety of different target cell types. Ad can accommodate up to 7.5 kb of exogenous genetic information. After Ad entry into the cells by way of specific receptors, the transferred genetic material is not inserted within the native cells' genome, thereby avoiding the development of insertional mutagenesis. The major disadvantage to this form of therapy is the humoral and cellular immune reactions that develop in response to the virus. This nonspecific inflammation may result in elimination of the target cell by immune mechanisms, thereby limiting the extent of transgene expression. Retroviruses contain a central core structure surrounding a viral RNA genome. A DNA polymerase (actually reverse transcriptase) converts the viral RNA into a DNA form. Upon entry into a cell nucleus, the DNA is randomly incorporated into the genome of the host cell, which imparts long-term expression. The use of retroviruses is limited because target cells must be replicating for the new gene to be incorporated into the genome, and random insertion creates the potential for insertional mutagenesis. AAV contains single-stranded DNA, which can accommodate cDNA. AAV is not pathogenic in humans, but does insert into the host genome randomly. Unlike the retroviruses, there is no need for cells to be actively dividing for efficient transduction.

IN VIVO ANGIOGENIC THERAPY FOR ISCHEMIC DISEASE

Several angiogenic molecules have been tested in animal models of ischemic tissue, including bFGF, aFGF, FGF-5, and VEGF isoforms. In some cases, the recombinant human protein was tested and in others, the naked DNA or adenoviral vectors were used. A single intra-arterial administration of 500 to 1000 µg of recombinant VEGF augmented perfusion and development of collateral vessels in a rabbit model of hindlimb ischemia.[24] Intramuscular or intra-arterial administration of aFGF, bFGF, HGF/SF,[10] and VEGF provided similar encouraging results.[25] Arterial gene transfer with cDNA encoding VEGF isoforms also led to revascularization to an extent comparable to that achieved with the recombinant protein. Calcium alginate capsules containing bFGF have been used to continuously deliver the growth factor to the heart over several weeks. This resulted in improved myocardial perfusion and contractility in the ischemic zone,[26] and normalization of endothelium-dependent relaxation of the collateral-dependent microcirculation.[27] Epicardial application of an aFGF mutant resulted in improved coronary blood flow, improved myocardial function, and normalized vasomotor regulation in the chronically ischemic territory.[28] In a pig model of coronary ischemia, minimal amounts of recombinant VEGF[29] or bFGF[26] delivered to periadventitial tissues resulted in a significant increase in coronary blood flow and functional improvement. Single intracoronary administration of these growth factors gave results similar to that of the 4-week infusion. Adenovirus-mediated gene transfer of VEGF or FGF-5 also resulted in collateral vessel growth and functional improvement in porcine models of myocardial ischemia.[30] These encouraging animal studies suggest that young, otherwise healthy animals are very responsive to exogenous growth factors in the context of ischemia.

Transmyocardial laser revascularization (TMR) is a relatively novel procedure in which transmural channels are created to presumably allow oxygenated ventricular blood to bathe the ischemic areas of myocardium. In 1933, myocardial sinusoids were identified in the human myocardium, which are believed to play a role in ventricular perfusion. In 1992, a 400-W carbon dioxide laser was used to revascularize a beating heart. In experimental models of canine heart ischemia, TMR has been found to increase tissue vascularity 2-fold to 3-fold and vascular cell proliferation by 8-fold. The mechanisms responsible for this increased vascularity within rat, porcine, and canine myocardium are thought to include angiogenesis, vascular remodeling, and vasculogenesis (de novo formation of blood vessels). Definitive evidence to support growth factor–mediated angiogenesis resulting from TMR has been provided by detailed immunohistochemical studies.[31] Results of clinical studies with TMR in humans show that it can decrease, but not eliminate the amount of myocardial ischemia. Improvement in blood flow is not immediate but may take between 3 and 6 months. Anatomical evidence of long-term channel patency has been provided at autopsy in patients who have had TMR. Patients who are poor candidates for conventional revascularization therapies such as percutaneous transluminal coronary angioplasty or coronary artery bypass grafting because of diffuse or small vessel disease may be ideal candidates for TMR. The promising clinical results, as demonstrated by improvement in angina class and exercise tolerance, are postulated to be secondary to a number of causes, including denervation, the establishment of patent blood vessels within the myocardium, and neovascularization through angiogenesis.

The successful augmentation of collateral vessel formation has been reported in a patient with peripheral vascular disease 4 weeks after direct intra-arterial gene transfer of a plasmid encoding VEGF.[32] In a study of 6 patients with thromboangiitis obliterans were treated with $phVEGF_{165}$ administered by direct intramuscular injection.[11] Gene expression was documented by assay of peripheral blood samples after the plasmid was administered. In 3 limbs, nonhealing ulcers were healed, and in 2 patients, ischemic rest pain was relieved. These authors suggest that gene transfer therapy, if instituted before the development of forefoot gangrene, could provide a therapeutic option for patients with advanced Buerger disease.[33] Cooke et al[34] reported their experience with intravenous administration of bFGF in a single patient with critical limb-threatening ischemia. This patient received bFGF 3 times a week for 6 weeks. A beneficial clinical response was detectable by week 4 of therapy, which was characterized by an improved walking distance, relief of ischemic pain, a marked reduction in analgesic consumption, and healing of persistent, unresponsive, painful inflammation of the hallux. The clinical improvement was sustained throughout the remaining weeks of therapy and follow-up evaluation. Plethysmography documented improved blood flow; specifically, the augmentation of digital flow was sustained and correlated with the marked improvement in the patient's clinical status. A phase I clinical trial of gene transfer by use of the naked plasmid DNA encoding for $VEGF_{165}$ was used in 10 patients with nonhealing ischemic ulcers. In these patients, the ankle-brachial index was significantly increased in the treated patients, and limb salvage was achieved in 3 patients who were to have lower extremity amputations.

Losordo et al[35] also used gene therapy in 5 patients who failed conventional therapy for coronary artery disease. These individuals were treated with naked plasmid DNA encoding $VEGF_{165}$, injected into the myocardium through a small lateral thoracotomy. All patients had a significant reduction in anginal symptoms, and postoperative ejection fractions were either unchanged or improved. In a clinical trial, patients undergoing coronary artery bypass grafting were given intramyocardial injections of FGF-1.[36]Those patients so treated were found to have evidence of distal neovascularization compared with controls. Selective imaging by intra-arterial subtraction angiography documented formation of new capillaries at injection sites. No adverse effects were observed. Based on these findings, the authors concluded that FGF-1 might be useful as adjunctive therapy to treat peripheral stenoses in the coronary circulation that cannot be revascularized surgically. Henry et al[37] showed that intracoronary infusion of VEGF markedly improved perfusion in one half of the patients, as demonstrated by thallium scintigraphy. In a phase I clinical trial, bFGF (FGF-2) protein was administered to nonbypassable regions of the heart during coronary bypass with the use of alginate polymer in 8 patients. After 3 months, treated patients had greater perfusion and myocardial function.[38] In a randomized, double-blind, placebo- controlled study using sustained release of FGF-2 by heparin alginate microcapsules in patients undergoing coronary bypass, all patients receiving high doses of FGF-2[13] were free from angina.[39] Stress nuclear perfusion imaging at baseline and 3 months after coronary artery bypass grafting showed a trend toward worsening of the defect size in the placebo group, and a significant reduction in the target tissue ischemic zone in the high-dose FGF-2 group. VEGF has been administered to the hearts of 21 patients by direct intramyocardial injection of the plasmid via an adenoviral vector as an adjunct to conventional coronary artery bypass grafting.[40,41] There were no reported systemic or cardiac-related adverse events related to vector administration. All patients reported improvement of anginal class after therapy. Coronary angiography and sestamibi scans demonstrated improvement of perfusion and ventricular wall function 30 days after therapy.

Therapeutic angiogenesis may be important in the management of peptic ulcer disease. Peptic ulcers in animals appear to be deficient in microvessels in the ulcer bed. In preclinical studies in which bFGF was orally administered to rats, the healing rate of duodenal ulcers was accelerated. In gastric ulcers in humans, levels of bFGF are substantially lower than in normal mucosa. Oral administration of the acid stable form of bFGF resulted in healing in ulcers caused by nonsteroidal anti-inflammatory drugs.

ANTIANGIOGENIC THERAPY: CLINICAL AND EXPERIMENTAL CONCEPTS

Several experimental studies suggest that primary tumor growth, invasiveness, and metastasis require neovascularization. A solid neoplasm is unable to grow beyond a critical volume without neovascularization.[42] Tumor-associated angiogenesis is a complex multistep process under the control of a variety of positive and negative stimuli. Tumor-associated endothelium is homogenous and divides up to 50 times more frequently than ECs of normal tissues, and may acquire the capability of secreting certain growth factors and cytokines that sustain its own growth (ie, autocrine regulation). Of the many known angiogenic proteins, those most commonly found in tumors appear to be bFGF and VEGF. The angiogenic phenotype may be the result of upregulation of ECGFs or downregulation of naturally occurring inhibitors of angiogenesis. Activated ECs are the primary target for inhibition of angiogenesis, and their therapeutic targeting presents several advantages over therapy directed against tumor cells. First, under physiologic conditions, endothelium is normally quiescent in normal adult tissues. This knowledge suggests that it may be possible to inhibit tumor vascularization selectively without affecting normal vasculature, thereby avoiding systemic adverse effects. Second, ECs are normal diploid and genetically stable cells, and therefore represent a uniform target as compared with tumor cells. Third, endothelium is a cellular target that can be easily reached by antiangiogenic agents administered systemically. In contrast, the activity of chemotherapeutic agents against tumors can be modulated by the blood supply, vascular architecture, and vascular permeability within solid tumors. Because of these factors, a steady stream of talented investigators have been seeking angiogenic inhibitors with the potential for widespread clinical use for nearly 3 decades. In the search for antiangiogenic compounds, it became clear that quantitation of angiogenesis in a biopsy specimen may predict the risk of metastasis or recurrence. Quantitation of microvessel density in breast cancer specimens has provided an indication of the risk of metastasis. A positive association between tumor angiogenesis and risk of metastasis, tumor recurrence, or death has been reported with regard to various other types of tumors.[43]

Angiogenic diseases occur in clinical conditions that do not involve neoplastic processes. Ocular neovascularization is a major cause of blindness worldwide. Various forms of retinal neovascularization in infants and adults are thought to be triggered by hypoxia in the area of the retina. Recent evidence suggests that VEGF is the chief mediator of this form of angiogenesis.[44] Neovascularization in atherosclerotic plaques may also be mediated by the overexpression of VEGF and by local hypoxia, and may contribute to growth and rupture of a plaque. In hemangiomas of infancy, VEGF and bFGF expression is excessive during the proliferative phase. Angiogenic factors released by macrophages, immune cells, and various inflammatory cells may mediate the ingrowth of a vascular pannus in rheumatoid joints. Elevated levels of VEGF have been detected in children with Crohn disease. Hypervascular skin lesions in patients with psoriasis overexpress the angiogenic polypeptide interleukin-8 and underexpress an inhibitor of angiogenesis, thrombospondin-1.[14] Dysfunction of endogenous angiogenic stimulators or inhibitors may underlie several female reproductive disorders such as prolonged menstrual bleeding and infertility. Developmental disorders such as bowel atresia, vascular malformations, hemangiomas, and unilateral facial atrophy may result from defects in angiogenesis or vasculogenesis.

One of the first inhibitors of angiogenesis was discovered in cartilage, a poorly vascularized tissue, by Brem and Folkman.[45] This agent could not be completely purified, making sufficient amounts unavailable for testing its antitumor activity. Protamine was found to have an angiosuppressive effect.[46] Protamine is a 4.3-kd, arginine-rich, cationic heparin-binding protein that inhibits EC migration and proliferation. It was later determined that certain steroids inhibit angiogenesis as well as some heparin-binding compounds. All of these agents were found to suppress neovascularization by altering the basement membrane turnover in growing blood vessels. In 1990, Ingber et al[47] noted fungal contamination in EC cultures causing a local gradient of EC rounding. From this seminal observation, fumagillin was isolated and purified from *Aspergillus fumigatus fresienus* and found to be a powerful angiosuppressive agent in vivo. The systemic toxicity associated with fumagillin resulted in testing of several analogues (such as TNP-470), the most potent being AGM-1470, which was found to be 50 times more active than the parent compound. AGM-1470 inhibits EC proliferation and prevents entry of ECs into the G1 phase of the cell cycle. Administration of TNP-470 to a rat model of spontaneous rheumatoid arthritis resulted in regression of the vascular pannus responsible for cartilage and joint destruction. Recent studies demonstrate that combined administration of AGM-1470 with other antiangiogenic agents, as well as with cytotoxic drugs or radiation therapy, enhances antitumor activity compared with the administration of each agent by itself. The work of D'Amato et al[48] recently showed that thalidomide, a sedative drug with teratogenic effects, was found to have moderate antiangiogenic effects. Interleukin-12 seems to have significant antiangiogenic activity, presumably by boosting host immunity and activating cytotoxic T lymphocytes. Transretinoic acid and its derivative appear to render ECs refractory to angiogenic stimuli and may also block secretion of growth factors by tumor cells in vitro. Another strategy to suppress angiogenesis is neutralization of specific angiogenic peptides. Monoclonal antibodies to bFGF and VEGF have been found to induce partial regression of solid tumors in vivo. Inhibitors of matrix metalloproteinases, important proteolytic enzymes that facilitate the invasiveness of tumor cells, induce tumor regression. A noncatalytic matrix metalloproteinase fragment with integrin-binding activity can regulate the invasive behavior of new blood vessels.

Two naturally occurring inhibitors of angiogenesis, angiostatin[49] and endostatin,[50] were recently sequenced. These molecules specifically inhibit proliferating and migrating blood vessels, but do not affect quiescent ECs. Angiostatin was purified as a 38-kd protein and is an internal fragment of human plasminogen. Human prostatic cancer cells release a substance with enzymatic activity that converts plasminogen to angiostatin. Systemic administration of recombinant angiostatin seems to maintain the dormancy of tumor metastases by enhancing the rate of apoptosis. Angiostatin was found to have no apparent systemic toxicity. Endostatin is a 20-kD C-terminal fragment of collagen XVIII that has been isolated from cultures of mouse hemangioendothelioma. Endostatin modulates apoptosis and is 30 times more potent than angiostatin. Apparently, resistance to endostatin has not been demonstrated in a variety of in vivo or in vitro models. Combination therapy with angiostatin and endostatin in mice bearing Lewis lung carcinoma resulted in complete tumor regression, whereas minimal disease was observed when single agents were used. This synergistic effect, combined with the complete absence of systemic toxicity and acquired resistance, suggests that these drugs may have the most clinically applicable promise for treatment of human cancers.

CLINICAL ANTIANGIOGENIC THERAPY

Hemangiomas occur in neonates and can grow rapidly in the first year of life. Approximately 10% of these hemangiomas cause serious damage, interfere with a vital organ, or become life threatening. Laboratory studies suggesting that interferon alfa-2a could be antiangiogenic led to its successful use in life-threatening pulmonary hemangioma in a 7-year old child.[51] Interferon alfa-2a suppresses the production of fibroblast growth factors from tumor cells, which probably accounts for the efficacy of the drug against these tumors. In a subsequent study of 20 neonates and infants with life-threatening or vision-threatening hemangiomas that failed to respond to corticosteroid therapy, most of the lesions regressed by 50% or more after 8 months of treatment. In a 5-year-old girl with a large recurrent giant cell tumor of the mandible, bFGF was found to be elevated in her urine.[52] The patient was treated with interferon alfa-2a for 1 year. After treatment, urinary bFGF levels decreased to normal and the tumor regressed. In a phase I clinical trial, TNP- 470, a new inhibitor of angiogenesis, was administered to patients with advanced squamous cell carcinoma of the uterine cervix. One woman who received this drug over 22 months had complete regression of the tumor, with no evidence of recurrent disease 8 months after it had been discontinued.[53] Three other patients in the trial had stable disease, whereas 14 had progressive disease. In another phase I trial of TNP-470, patients with AIDS-related Kaposi sarcoma received the drug for 24 weeks. Tumor responses were observed in a number of patients, at a variety of dosages; the median duration to the response was 11 weeks.[54] In another study, TNP-470 was administered to patients with advanced cancer, refractory to all conventional therapies. Principal toxicities included dizziness, lightheadedness, vertigo, ataxia, anxiety, and depression. The pharmokinetic evaluations in this study suggested that the short plasma half-life warranted prolonged intravenous infusion.[55] Agents that neutralize growth factors, such as bFGF and VEGF, have been entered into clinical trials. Anti-VEGF antibodies have completed phase I clinical trials designed to evaluate systemic toxicity. Based on minimal toxicity, phase II and III trials are planned for refractory tumors. Substances known to interfere with VEGF-mediated receptor signal transduction have been entered into clinical trials. More than 10 antiangiogenesis agents (including angiostatin and endostatin) are currently in clinical trials. The results of these trials will have substantial impact on therapeutic strategies for a variety of disease processes.

FUTURE HORIZONS AND SUMMARY

Angiogenic therapies for ischemic, malignant, and benign proliferative diseases carry tremendous clinical promise. There is a broad mandate for angiogenic therapies to address a variety of disease processes, extending from cancer to atherosclerosis. Inhibitors of angiogenesis are cytostatic agents that need proper clinical evaluation, and development of biological markers to confirm their biological activity. Efficient delivery of angiogenic therapies directly to the target tissue is essential to obtain the best biological response. Once phase I studies have identified agents with an acceptable toxicologic profile, future research will include evaluations of combined therapeutic agents. A similar approach (ie, to evaluate combined pharmacologic agents) will be required in the development of angiogenic approaches to ameliorate ischemic syndromes involving myocardium or skeletal muscle. As angiogenic (or antiangiogenic) agents become available for widespread use, it is unclear to what extent classic surgical interventions (excisions, bypass surgery) may contribute to treating the underlying clinical problem.

REFERENCES

1. Folkman J, Cole P, Zimmerman S: Tumor behaviour in isolated perfused organs. *Ann Surg* 164:491-502, 1966.
2. Pardanuad L, Yassine F, Dieterlen-Lievre F: Relationship between vasculogenesis, angiogenesis and hematopoiesis during avian ontogeny. *Development* 105:473-485, 1989.
3. Hobson B, Denekamp J: Endothelial proliferation in tumors and normal tissues: Continuous labelling studies. *Br J Cancer* 49:405-413, 1984.
4. Gimbrone M, Cotran R, Leapman S, et al: Tumor growth and neovascularization: An experimental model using the rabbit cornea. *J Natl Cancer Inst* 52:413-427, 1974.
5. Klagsbrun M, Knighton D, Folkman J: Tumor angiogenesis activity in cells grown in tissue culture. *Cancer Res* 36:110-114, 1976.
6. Birdwell C, Gospodarwowicz G, Nicolson G: Factors from 3T3 cells stimulate proliferation of cultured vascular endothelial cells. *Nature* 268:528-531, 1977.
7. Gimbrone M, Cotran R, Folkman J: Endothelial regeneration: Studies with human endothelial cells in culture. *Ser Haematol* 6:453-455, 1973.

8. Folkman J, Haudenschild C, Zetter B: Long term culture of capillary endothelial cells. *Proc Natl Acad Sci U S A* 76:5217-5221, 1979.

9. Gospadarowicz D, Bialecki H, Greenburg G: Purification of the fibroblast growth factor activity from bovine brain. *J Biol Chem* 253:3736-3743, 1978.

10. Maciag T, Cerundolo I, Kelley P, et al: An endothelial cell growth factor from bovine hypothalamus: Identification and partial characterization. *Proc Natl Acad Sci U S A* 76:5674-5678, 1979.

11. D'Amore P, Glaser B, Brunson S, et al: Angiogenic activity from bovine retina: Partial purification and characterization. *Proc Natl Acad Sci USA* 78:3068, 1981.

12. Barritault D, Arruti C, Courtois Y: Is there a ubiquitous growth factor in the eye? Proliferation induced in different cell types by eye derived growth factors. *Differentiation* 18:29-42, 1981.

13. Klagsbrun M, Smith S: Purification of a cartilage- derived growth factor. *J Biol Chem* 255:10859-10866, 1980.

14. Shing Y, Folkman J, Sullivan R, et al: Heparin affinity: Purification of a tumor-derived capillary endothelial cell growth factor. *Science* 223:1296, 1984.

15. Esch F, Baird A, Ling N, et al: Primary structure of bovine pituitary basic fibroblast growth factor and comparison with the amino-terminal sequence of bovine brain acidic FGF. *Proc Natl Acad Sci U S A* 82:6507-6511, 1985.

16. Thomas K, Rios-Candelore M, Giminez-Gallegos G, et al: Pure brain-derived acidic fibroblast growth factor is a potent angiogenic vascular endothelial cell mitogen with sequence homology to interleukin 1. *Proc Natl Acad Sci U S A* 82:6409-6413, 1985.

17. Burgess W, Maciag T: The heparin-binding (fibroblast) growth factor family of proteins. *Ann Rev Biochem* 58:575-606, 1989.

18. Carreira C, LaVallee T, Tarantini F, et al: S100A13 is involved in the regulation of fibroblast growth factor-1 and p40 synaptotagmin-1 release in vitro. *J Biol Chem* 273:22224-22231, 1998.

19. Ferrara N, Henzel W: Pituitary follicular cells secrete a novel heparin binding growth factor specific for vascular endothelial cells. *Biochem Biophys Res Commun* 161:851-858, 1989.

20. Leung D, Cachianes G, Kuang W, et al: Vascular endothelial cell growth factor is a secreted angiogenic mitogen. *Science* 246:1306-1309, 1989.

21. Ferrara N, Carver Moore K, Chen H, et al: Heterozygous embryonic lethality induced by targeted inactivation of the VEGF gene. *Nature* 380:439-442, 1996.

22. Pepper M, Ferrara N, Orci L, et al: Potent synergism between vascular endothelial cell growth factor and basic fibroblast growth factor in the induction of angiogenesis in vitro. *Biochem Biophys Res Commun* 189:824-831, 1992.

23. Pepper M, Ferrara N, Orci L, et al: Vascular endothelial growth factor (VEGF) induces plasminogen activators and plasminogen activator

inhibitor-1 in microvascular endothelial cells. *Biochem Biophys Res Commun* 181:902-906, 1991.

24. Takeshita S: Therapeutic angiogenesis: A single intra- arterial bolus of vascular endothelial cell growth factor augments revascularization in a rabbit ischemic hind limb model. *J Clin Invest* 93:662-670, 1994.

25. Witzenblicher B: Vascular endothelial cell growth factor-C (VEGF-C/VEGF-2) promotes angiogenesis in the setting of tissue ischemia. *Am J Path*ol 153:381-394, 1998.

26. Harada K, Grossman W, Friedman M: Basic fibroblast growth factor improves myocardial function in chronically ischemic porcine hearts. *J Clin Invest* 94:623-630, 1994.

27. Sellke F, Wang S, Friedman M, et al: Basic FGF enhances endothelium-dependent relaxation of the collateral-perfused coronary microcirculation. *Am J Physiol* 267:H1303-1311, 1994.

28. Sellke F, Li J, Stamler A, et al: Angiogenesis induced by acidic fibroblast growth factor as an alternative method of revascularization for chronic myocardial ischemia. *Surgery* 120:182-188, 1996.

29. Pearlman J: Magnetic resonance mapping demonstrates benefits of VEGF-induced myocardial angiogenesis. *Nat Med* 1:1085- 1089, 1995.

30. Giordano F, Pina P, McKirnan MD, et al: Intracoronary gene transfer of fibroblast growth factor-5 increases blood flow and contractile function in an ischemic region of the heart. *Nat Med* 2:534-539, 1996.

31. Pelletier M, Giaid A, Sivaraman S, et al: Angiogenesis and growth factor expression in a model of transmyocardial revascularization. *Ann Thorac Surg* 66:12-18, 1998.

32. Isner J, Pieczek A, Schainfeld R, et al: Clinical evidence of angiogenesis after arterial gene transfer of phVEGF165 in patient with ischemic limb. *Lancet* 348:370-374, 1996.

33. Isner JM, Baumgartner I, Rauh G, et al: Treatment of thromboangiitis obliterans (Buerger's disease) by intramuscular gene transfer of vascular endothelial growth factor: Preliminary clinical results. *J Vasc Surg* 28:964-973, 1998.

34. Cooke JP, Bhatnagar R, Szuba A, et al: Fibroblast growth factor as therapy for critical limb ischemia: A case report. *Vasc Med* 4:89-91, 1999.

35. Losordo DW, Vale PR, Isner JM: Gene therapy for myocardial angiogenesis. *Am Heart J* 138:132-141, 1999.

36. Schumacher B, Pecher P, Von Spect B, et al: Induction of neoangiogenesis in ischemic myocardium by human growth factors: First clinical results of a new treatment of coronary heart disease. *Circulation* 97:645-650, 1998.

37. Henry T, Rocha-Singh K, Isner J, et al: Results of intracoronary recombinant human vascular endothelial cell growth factor (rhVEGF) administration trial. J Am Coll Cardiol 31:65A, 1998.

38. Sellke FW, Laham RJ, Edelman ER, et al: Therapeutic angiogenesis with basic fibroblast growth factor: Technique and early results. Ann Thorac Surg 65:1540-1544, 1998.

39. Laham R, Sellke F, Edelman E, et al: Local perivascular delivery of

basic fibroblast growth factor in patients undergoing coronary bypass surgery: Results of a phase I randomized, double-blind, placebo controlled trial. Circulation 100:1865-1871, 1999.

40. Rosengart TK, Lee LY, Patel SR, et al: Six-month assessment of a phase I trial of angiogenic gene therapy for the treatment of coronary artery disease using direct intramyocardial administration of an adenovirus vector expressing the VEGF121 cDNA. Ann Surg 230:466-470, 1999.

41. Rosengart TK, Lee LY, Patel SR, et al: Angiogenesis gene therapy: Phase I assessment of direct intramyocardial administration of an adenovirus vector expressing VEGF121 cDNA to individuals with clinically significant severe coronary artery disease. Circulation 100:468-474, 1999.

42. Folkman J: What is the evidence that tumors are angiogenesis dependent? J Natl Cancer Inst 82:4-6, 1989.

43. Weidner N: Intratumor microvessel density as a prognostic factor in cancer. Am J Pathol 147:9-19, 1995.

44. Miller J, Adamis A, Shima D, et al: Vascular endothelial growth factor/vascular permeability factor is temporally and spatially correlated with ocular angiogenesis in a primate model. Am J Pathol 145:574-584, 1994.

45. Brem H, Folkman J: Inhibition of tumor angiogenesis mediated by cartilage. J Exp Med 141:427-439, 1975.

46. Taylor S, Folkman J: Protamine is an inhibitor of angiogenesis. Nature 297:307-312, 1982.

47. Ingber D, Fujita T, Kishimoto S, et al: Synthetic analogues of fumagillin that inhibit angiogenesis and suppress tumor growth. Nature 348:555-557, 1990.

48. D'Amato RJ, Loughan MS, Flynn E, et al: Thalidomide is an inhibitor of angiogenesis. *Proc Natl Acad Sci USA* 91:4082-4084, 1994.

49. O'Reilly M, Holmgren L, Shing Y, et al: Angiostatin: A novel angiogenesis inhibitor that mediates the suppression of metastases by a Lewis lung carcinoma. Cell 79:315-328, 1994.

50. O'Reilly M, Boehm T, Shing Y, et al: Endostatin: An endogenous inhibitor of angiogenesis and tumor growth. Cell 88:277-285, 1997.

51. White C, Sondheimer H, Crouch E, et al: Treatment of pulmonary hemangiomatosis with recombinant interferon alpha-2a. N Engl J Med 320:1197-1200, 1989.

52. Kaban L, Mulliken J, Ezekowitz R, et al: Antiangiogenic therapy of a recurrent giant cell tumor of the mandible with interferon alfa-2a. Pediatrics 103:1145-1149, 1999.

53. Kudelka A, Verschragen C, Loyer E: Complete remission of metastatic cervical cancer with the angiogenesis inhibitor TNP-470. N Engl J Med 338:991-992, 1998.

54. Dezube B, Von Roenn J, Holden-Wiltse J, et al: Fumagillin analog in the treatment of Kaposi sarcoma: A phase I AIDS Clinical Trial Group Study. J Clin Oncol 146:1444-1449, 1998.

55. Bhargava P, Marshall J, Rizvi N, et al: A phase I and pharmokinetic study of TNP-470 administered weekly to patients with advanced cancer. Clin Cancer Res 5:1989-1995, 1999.

Index

A

Abciximab, in carotid stenting, 24, 25

Access
- arterial
  - bleeding after, management, 113-121
  - complications from, iatrogenic, management, 111-124
  - embolization after, management, 122
  - fistula after, arteriovenous, management, 122
  - infection after, management, 122
  - nerve injury during, management, 123
  - route of, 111-113
  - thrombosis after, management, 122
  - transfemoral, 111-112
  - upper extremity, 112-113
- for carotid angioplasty and stenting (*see* Carotid, angioplasty and stenting, access for)
- hemodialysis (*see* Hemodialysis, access)
- sites, vascular, impact of graft surveillance on longevity of, 161-168

Acetylsalicylic acid (*see* Aspirin)

Age, and complications of carotid angioplasty and stenting, 3

AGM-1470, 226

AIDS-related Kaposi's sarcoma, TNP-470 in, 227

Ambulatory status, before and after limb salvage surgery, 104

Amplatz wire, in carotid stenting, 13

Anesthesia, for carotid angioplasty and stenting, 7

Aneurysm, abdominal aortic
- animal models, 202-203
- infrarenal neck in, "long", angiogram of anatomy of, 68
- juxtarenal
  - patient demographics, 35
  - renal artery occlusive disease and, severe, 37
  - view of, 36
- matrix metalloproteinases in, 201-203
  - future direction, 203
- pararenal, repair of, 33-51
  - analysis, 44-50
  - literature summary, 47-48
  - operative data, 39
  - operative results, 41
  - operative technique, 38-41
  - outcome, 41-44
  - patients in study, 35-38
  - renal function data in, 38
- proteolysis in, 202
- ruptured
  - endovascular grafts for (*see* Endovascular grafts for abdominal aortic aneurysms, ruptured)
  - new treatment approach, 64
- suprarenal
  - patient demographics, 35
  - views of, anterior and oblique, 36

Angioaccess-induced steal syndrome (*see* Steal syndrome, ischemic, hemodialysis access-related)

Angiogenesis
- definition, 216
- regulation of, 215-231
- study techniques, 216